STEM CELLS - LABORATORY AND CLINICAL RESEARCH

CONCEPTS OF PERIODONTAL REGENERATION AND REGENERATIVE MEDICINE

MECHANISMS THAT MODULATE CELLS AND MATRICES

STEM CELLS – LABORATORY AND CLINICAL RESEARCH

Additional books in this series can be found on Nova's website under the Series tab.

Additional e-books in this series can be found on Nova's website under the e-book tab.

STEM CELLS - LABORATORY AND CLINICAL RESEARCH

CONCEPTS OF PERIODONTAL REGENERATION AND REGENERATIVE MEDICINE

MECHANISMS THAT MODULATE CELLS AND MATRICES

MENA SOORY

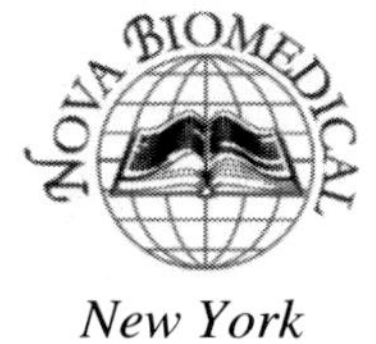

New York

Library of Congress Cataloging-in-Publication Data

Library of Congress Control Number: 2015940914

ISBN: 978-1-63482-970-0

Published by Nova Science Publishers, Inc. † New York

Contents

Preface		**vii**
Abstract		**ix**
Chapter 1	Introduction	**1**
Chapter 2	Strategies for Periodontal Regeneration	**5**
Chapter 3	Biomarkers of Cell Differentiation and Growth Promoting Agents	**17**
Chapter 4	Periosteal Cell Sheets and Tissue Matrix	**21**
Chapter 5	Functions of Hydrogels in Tissue Regeneration	**25**
Chapter 6	Regenerative Medicine, Cell Signalling and Gene Delivery	**33**
Chapter 7	Biomechanics of Stem Cells and Their Applications	**37**
Chapter 8	Smart Biomaterials and Scaffolds	**43**
Chapter 9	The Role of MicroRNAs in Tissue Engineering	**49**
Chapter 10	Three Dimensional (3D) Printing of Tissue Regenerative Materials and Their Applications	**61**
Conclusion		**67**
References		**69**
Index		**89**

Preface

There is a constant search for consistent, robust regenerative strategies, despite diverse methods and biomaterials that have enhanced tissue engineering technology over the decades; for improved healing potential in periodontal bone defects, applicable to regenerative medicine. They include regenerative surgical procedures, using a spectrum of biomimetics, growth factors and matrices. Replication of biologically effective functional tissue is an elusive goal.

The subject covers the principles of periodontal regeneration and strategies for tissue regenerative procedures encompassing materials, methods, and mechanisms involved; focused on the current status and future directions applicable to regenerative Medicine and Dentistry. Suitable targets for effective patient outcome are covered. They include cell-based and gene-based therapies with emphasis on interactions between cellular and matrix components. The approach is multi-disciplinary, combining the applications of bioengineering, molecular biology, material science and nanotechnology for coordination of repair and regeneration of lost or missing tissue.

The content embraced is applicable to a larger audience; providing insight into mechanisms involved; and greater potential for developing translational regenerative medicine with improved choices for predictability and consistency of applications. Multidisciplinary coverage of scientific content illustrates clinical applications of principles and mechanisms involved. It encompasses a range of biomedical approaches suitable for scientists interested in concepts of tissue regeneration and clinicians who wish to develop the strategies covered. Proof of principle coverage of clinical applications, provides potential for developing enhanced materials and methods of delivery, for a more consistent clinical outcome.

The content would be useful to scientists, dental and medical graduates/postgraduates with an interest in regenerative Medicine/Dentistry. It encompasses multidisciplinary content including biomedical concepts of tissue engineering and their applications. The academic level is suitable for scientists, dental and medical graduates/postgraduates with an interest in tissue engineering and regeneration of lost/missing tissues.

I would like to acknowledge my co-workers for their contribution to publications cited in the text.

Author:
Dr. Mena Soory
Periodontology
King's College London Dental Institute
Denmark Hill, London SE5 9RW
UK (Clinical academic)
Email: mena.soory@kcl.ac.uk

Abstract

Regenerative medicine and dentistry combine applications of molecular biology, material science, bioengineering and nanoscience in order to repair, regenerate and replace missing tissue. Diverse technologies have emerged in recent times to streamline applications of more predictable materials and methods; in order to attain the elusive goal of periodontal regeneration. In addition to grafting materials and barrier membranes to exclude epithelial downgrowth and promote mesenchymal elements, the environment of the cell is pivotal to events that follow. These include cell-based-, gene-based, protein and peptide therapy, application of scaffolds, lasers, harnessing bone anabolic activity and the resolution of inflammation. Recommendations embrace suitable targets for patient outcome, based on clinical applications of scientific principles for more predictable and consistent results, in regenerating hard and soft tissues of a functional periodontium.

Various approaches have evolved, including autologous tissue, growth factors, platelet concentrates and scaffolds. Appropriate manipulation of stem cells using sophisticated technology, makes them versatile for a range of applications. Decellularised extracellular matrices containing a complex assembly of relevant growth factors, matrix macromolecules and fibrillar proteins that mimic the natural ECM; have significant biomedical applications for coating scaffolds, as adhesive cell culture substrates and tissue engineered products. Interactions of extracellular vesicles (EV) with ECM/relevant cells, affect cell signalling, differentiation and proliferation. This has potential for the development of a focal cell phenotype with applications in regenerative medicine; including stem-cell based therapeutic interventions. Incorporation of EV in regenerative therapy, includes combination with hydrogels and applications for scaffold coatings, by linking with cell- and ECM-interactive fibrin gels.

The endogenous, highly conserved small, non-coding microRNA molecules, have applications in regulating post-transcriptional gene expression by binding to their target mRNAs. Periosteal cell sheets are effective in enhancing bone formation. Autologous cell sheets are readily translated for clinical applications. Endothelial and mesenchymal 3D printing have evolved as the cutting edge of tissue engineering research. 3D printing enables the synthesis of multi-material and cell-laden biomimetic and nanostructured scaffolds more effectively, with less effort. These concepts are reviewed in the context of a coordinated strategy for effective combinations to deliver more consistent applications and outcome.

Chapter 1

Introduction

Regenerative medicine combines applications of molecular biology, material science, bioengineering, nanoscience and biomaterials in order to repair, regenerate and replace missing tissue [1]. Various approaches have evolved, including autologous tissue, growth factors, platelet concentrates and scaffolds. The use of adult stem cells overcomes ethical problems. Appropriate manipulation of stem cells using sophisticated technology, makes them versatile for a range of applications. These perspectives offer accessible sources that are rich in mesenchymal stem cells, including the oral cavity, thus minimizing morbidity. Initial stem cell-lines as a starting point, in combination with principles of nanotechnology and innovative scaffolds, have potential for regeneration of lost tissue and organ systems comprising multiple tissues. Decellularised extracellular matrices (ECM) have extensive applications in the field of cell biology, tissue engineering and regenerative medicine. Cell-derived matrices comprise a complex assembly of relevant growth factors, matrix macromolecules and fibrillar proteins that mimic the natural ECM [2]. They have significant biomedical applications for coating scaffolds, as adhesive cell culture substrates and tissue engineered products; and are at a relatively early stage of development, requiring further progression. Their applications, current limitations and future directions are reviewed.

Extracellular vesicles (EV) are exosomes resulting from fusion of microvesicular components with the cell membrane from which they are released directly [3]. EV are involved in diverse aspects of cell activity including intercellular signalling, cell differentiation and proliferation, applicable to regenerative medicine. Restoration of tissue resulting from organ damage is one of the paracrine applications of EV in stem-cell based therapeutic interventions. These actions are harnessed in the paracrine modulation of cell recruitment, differentiation, proliferation and angiogenesis relevant to tissue engineering. Incorporation of EV in regenerative therapy includes combination with hydrogels, co-injection and EV scaffold coatings by linking with fibrin gels, interactive with cells and ECM. ECM plays a major role in providing guidance for cellular interaction, strength and form to newly synthesized tissue, fundamental to tissue engineering. The molecular composition and structure of ECM determine cell recruitment, differentiation and their sustenance for a focal cell phenotype to develop. Strategies for biodegradable scaffolds with load bearing and cell retentive functions, need to be complemented and sustained by locally produced ECM, following scaffold degradation. Interactions of EV with ECM-producing cells or direct influences on ECM affect their composition. They show great potential for therapeutics, biomarker research and also provide alternatives to stem cell based approaches associated with paracrine effects. There is great promise for the applications of engineered EV to support endogenous repair and enhance existing approaches to regenerative Medicine and Dentistry.

Considering the sensitivity of cells and tissues to the ambient microenvironment in regenerative medicine, diverse strategies have been used to create suitable niches for cell proliferation, renewal and enhancement of appropriate fate of cell differentiation. In order to mimic *in vivo* conditions *in vitro*, several biomimetic conditions have evolved, to regulate cell phenotype and functions [4]. A computer-assisted design/manufacturing technology utilizing 3D photolithography is an innovative method with versatile biomedical applications. It is used for the fabrication of nanostructured and biomimetic scaffolds with applications in regenerative medicine and tissue engineering.

Despite the capacity of tissue for self-repair and regeneration, complex pathology or trauma could contribute to its deficit, affecting the quality of life of individuals. Diverse treatment strategies are used to overcome tissue deficit, including complex grafting methods. Autografts may not be widely used, due to limited supply and morbidity of donor sites. Allografts and xenografts overcome some of these problems, however transmission of infectious diseases would be a concern. In view of these limitations, current advances provide innovative approaches for tissue engineering using bioactive growth factor delivery and cell-matrix interactions with effectively designed scaffolds [5]. A combination of progenitor cells seeded in biocompatible scaffolds with suitable bioconductive agents such as growth factors is fundamental to bone/tissue engineering. Effective cell based therapies coordinate regulatory activity of cell-signalling molecules, cells and intercellular matrices. Approaches including cell expansion in hypoxic conditions for maintenance of pluripotency, cell differentiation for autologous therapies, regulation of RANKL and growth factor expression; have been explored in regenerative medicine. Refinement of scaffolds that take their cues from extracellular matrix is an important aspect of bone tissue engineering.

Polycaprolactone-colactide scaffolds that are coated with collagen/chondroitin sulphate are effective in enhancing *de novo* bone formation. Improved mechanical strength, apatite mineralization, biocompatibility and good drug delivery are associated with nanosized, mesoporous, glass/poly (lactic-co-glycolic acid) composite coated CaSiO3 scaffolds that are multifunctional [6] and show promise for bone engineering. By changing the internal phase of microparticles, drug loading efficacy and release profiles are enhanced. These concepts provide a better understanding of drug release characteristics of scaffolds for future clinical applications. Cell adhesion could be affected by substrate preference properties of biomaterials. Hydrogels have useful applications in regenerative Medicine/Dentistry. The effects of cyclical tensile strain on differentiation of cells towards an osteogenic lineage have been evaluated [7], to clarify concepts of strain-induced bone remodelling. There are multidisciplinary contributions to the field of bone tissue engineering, which continue to evolve in their expertise independently; and depict current trends for wider applications in medical and dental specialties. These trends are addressed in greater detail in the chapters that follow.

Chapter 2

Strategies for Periodontal Regeneration

Periodontal disease is initiated by plaque biofilm, leading to compromised bone support of teeth. It results in eventual tooth loss if left untreated. Current treatment methods are effective in controlling active periodontal disease; while regeneration of the supporting structures of teeth remains an elusive goal. The ultimate objective of periodontal regeneration is the formation of new cementum, supportive periodontal ligament and bone. Current therapies lack consistency in achieving this goal in a predictable way. Periodontal regeneration requires appropriate sequencing of regulatory signals, availability of progenitor cells, extracellular matrix and adequate vasculature. The regenerative process may be regulated by modulating signalling pathways of relevant molecules, cells or the extracellular matrix and scaffolds. Bone marrow mesenchymal stem cells provide tremendous potential in regenerative medicine. High quality regenerative tissue formation is one of the advantages of using mesenchymal stem cell progenitors, with minimal morbidity at the donor site. It is significant that gingival tissue-derived mesenchymal stem cells are a readily accessible source of autografts, with a low risk of immune rejection. The main tissue sources of mesenchymal stem cells in the oral cavity and their applications in regenerative therapy are reviewed; particularly, gingival tissue-derived mesenchymal stem cells which are readily accessed. Their induction into osteogenic, chondrogenic and adipogenic lineages has been evaluated [8].

Diverse technologies have emerged in recent times to enhance opportunities for reaching the elusive goal of periodontal regeneration. In addition to grafting materials and barrier membranes to exclude epithelium and promote mesenchymal elements, the environmental envelope of the cell is pivotal to events that follow. A consensus view on the goal for hard and soft tissue reconstruction of the periodontium has been developed, based on a workshop on periodontal regeneration. Emerging ideas and reference points are prioritized for future development [9]. These include cell-based, gene-based, protein and peptide therapy, application of scaffolds, lasers; harnessing bone anabolic activity, resolution of inflammation and effects of the microbiome. Recommendations embrace suitable target cells for patient outcome based on clinical applications of scientific principles. They provide more predictable and consistent results, in regenerating hard and soft tissues of a functional periodontium; within safety requirements and an effective cost/benefit ratio.

Progression of chronic inflammatory periodontitis leads to loss of the supporting structures of teeth, comprising periodontal ligament, alveolar bone and root cementum, resulting in tooth loss. There have been several attempts at regenerating complex periodontal tissues. As a result, a useful experimental model has evolved for the provision of future regenerative therapies [10], with more sustained and comprehensive restoration of lost tissue. Guided bone/tissue regeneration utilizes a range of growth factors, grafts and synthetic substitutes as drivers of endogenous regenerative mechanisms initiated by recruitment of host cells; and the application of stem cell therapeutics for enhanced periodontal tissue regeneration with biological integration. Supplementation of these approaches with other methods provides a more consistent strategy in this context. The delivery, efficacy, safety and applications of current stem cell based approaches for periodontal regeneration and their future applications are addressed. Considering the limitations of current barrier memebranes for guided tissue regeneration, a degradable material comprising a composite of polylactic acid and nanohydroxyapatite (nHA-PLA) was assessed; for its capacity as a bioactive material and as a carrier for growth factors, using PDGF [11]. There was active delivery of PDGF and improved cell differentiation at higher nHA levels. Bone regeneration and biodelivery of active molecules are enhanced in nHA-PLA composite material containing a high concentration of nHA, in addition to its barrier function.

Periodontal regenerative strategies are based on embryonic mechanisms; the formation of root cementum being a critical element in regeneration of the periodontium [12]. The Hertwig's epithelial root sheath (HERS) plays a pivotal role in root formation and cementogenesis, although traditionally, the origin of cementoblast differentiation has been attributed to ectomesenchymal cells of the dental follicle. Regenerative therapy aims to focus on regeneration of lost periodontal tissue towards a functional periodontium using guided tissue regeneration and biological agents such as enamel matrix derivative. Residual elements of HERS persisting in the periodontal ligament as the epithelial cell rests of Malassez are considered to be a stem cell niche for new cementoblasts. Cementoblast differentiation has been attributed to enamel matrix protein and members of the transforming growth factor- β (TGF-β) superfamily. Lost periodontal tissue as a result of periodontitis may be regenerated with improved therapies, based on knowledge of intercellular communication for the differentiation of cementoblasts.

The dental apical papilla (DAP) is a less well documented source of MSCs, in addition to dental pulp and periodontal ligament. It presents an accessible source, for cell-based therapies and procedures for tissue engineering. Implantation of MSCs results in trophic-mediated repair and regeneration with a signalling circuit that promotes these actions. As TGF-β is an important growth factor associated with tissue regeneration and repair, it is hypothesized that microenvironmental cues could induce the production and secretion of TGF-β in DAP-derived MSCs [13]. When these cells (hSCAPs) are encapsulated in diverse matrices for the evaluation of TGF-β3 secretion, there are dynamic changes in mechanical stress and cell-matrix interaction sensed by the cells in culture; during their transition from a monolayer culture (2-dimensional) towards a 3-D culture environment, rather than the chemical composition of the scaffold influencing the synthesis and release of TGF-β3. It is relevant that there is a 10-fold less secretion of TGF-β3 in monolayer cultures. These interactions are a cornerstone for the development of more effective strategies pertaining to cell therapy and tissue engineering for the reconstruction of lost tissue in a more consistent manner.

Recent advances in regenerative technologies comprising matrix scaffolds, cell/gene therapy and drug delivery biologics; for enhanced reconstruction of bone defects associated with teeth and implants, have been reviewed [14]. Criteria for optimizing scaffold design, to regenerate functional tissues with a physiological role have been appraised. Pre-clincial and clinical studies have been assessed throughout, for the scope of growth factors and allied agents, advances in stem cell and gene therapy; and novel developments for enhanced regulation of spatiotemporal release kinetics of growth factors, from improved matrix-based delivery platforms. Current limitations drive progressive work, towards the development of predictable reproducibility of functional osseous tissue. The biomimetic properties and regenerative potential of scaffold-based delivery platforms, for cells and growth promoting agents; hold promise for targeted therapy focused on more predicatable patient outcome.

The commonest diseases leading to tooth and tissue loss are periodontal disease and dental caries. Consequently, applications for tissue engineering and regenerative dental needs are documented. There are several sources of somatic stem cells from teeth and the periodontium for tissue regeneration. Self-assembled biomimetic peptides, 3D printing and microfabrication are novel trends in biomaterial science with potential for regeneration of teeth and lost tissues of the periodontium, for sustenance of health and functionality [15]. A combination of scaffolds, stem cells, tissue culture, growth factors, grafting and transplantation drive the creation of contructs for tissue regeneration [16]. The clinical outcome of these procedures is affected by diverse subject variables associated with disease susceptibility and response to treatment which would affect consistency.

Periodontal regeneration is enhanced by barrier membrane technology, stimulatory proteins for cell growth and gene delivery. Diverse cells of periodontal origin are influenced by factors that contribute to differentiation and development of connective tissue and bone. Attenuation of current strategies in a milieu of inflammatory periodontitis is a limitation that needs to be overcome, for optimal efficacy of proposed agents and mechanisms thereof. Pleiotropic actions of soluble molecular signals closely regulate epithelial/mesenchymal interactions in mineralized and non-mineralized tissues. Molecular redundancy associated with multiple isoforms poses a challenge for focused delivery of components required for periodontal regeneration. Fine-tuned, streamlined activity of redundant isoforms of human osteogenic proteins is a significant advance in regenerative tissue engineering; underscored by accurate dissemination of active agents to connective tissue and bone. These concepts have been reviewed, including recent patents on the subject [17]. Critical temporal phases of wound healing are regulated by targeted therapy comprising loaded scaffolds, fillers, vehicular microcapsules and slow release devices for the delivery of stimulatory agents. Tissue engineering techniques and gene therapy enhance expansion of cell populations and protein expression. Targeted delivery of growth stimulatory agents via scaffolds, barriers, cell sheets and their variants, would pave the way for future applications in human subjects, with more consistent outcome.

Management of periodontal intrabony defects is an important therapeutic goal. The efficacy of available approaches for their treatment outcome and strategy for future work are defined [18]. A systematic review based on searches in PubMed and Cochrane databases supplemented by original reports and reviews focus on proof of principle histological evidence of periodontal regeneration, clinical trials and case reports. The primary outcome variable was considered to be a change in intrabony defect fill and the secondary outcome was a change in clinical attachment, for analytical purposes. The quality and strength of evidence was evaluated using the SORT (Strength of Recommendation Taxonomy) grade. The quality, quantity and consistency of evidence are addressed in order to provide a rating of individual studies. It is built around a framework with emphasis on measuring changes in morbidity and mortality related to patient-orientated outcome measures [19]. Evaluation of the use of biologics in periodontal regeneration showed that enamel matrix derivative (EMD) and recombinant human platelet derived growth factor (rhPDGF-BB) with β-tricalcium phosphate (β-TCP) were effective in regenerating intrabony defects. Numerous studies support the level of evidence for efficacy of these materials; showing improved clinical attachment on previously diseased root surfaces, decreased probing pocket depths, gain in radiographic bone levels and improved periodontal health. It is comparable to certain bone replacement grafts and guided tissue regeneration (GTR), maintained over prolonged periods of greater than 10 years. These findings are consistent with available histological evidence.

Enamel matrix derivative (EMD), is a viable option for regenerating lost tissues of the periodontium. Its active component is derived from foetal porcine enamel extract, prepared commercially. Complex interactions with host cells mimicking odontogenesis have attracted considerable interest in researching its actions and applications. The composition and mechanisms of action of amelogenin and ameloblastin, the components of EMD, including effects on diverse cell types *in vitro* have been reviewed [20]. A functional model involving nanosphere formation, aggregation and dissolution is presented for EMD. By using current knowledge on the structure, constitution and regulation of its actions, there is improved understanding of its regenerative mechanisms, enabling a defined functional model of EMD for its applications and cell /tissue interactions. Greater than 90% of its composition comprises amelogenin proteins as the dominant protein complex, including alternatively spliced and enzymically cleaved components; with relatively small amounts of ameloblastin. EMD has significant effects on angiogenesis, gene expression, cell proliferation and differentiation in cells of the periodontal ligament and osteoblastic lineage. Conversely cytostatic effects of EMD on epithelial cells, impair their activity. The leucine-rich amelogenin peptide has similar effects, but to a lesser degree. Both the amelogenin and ameloblastin peptides demonstrate osteogenic effects. Synergistic actions between cells and diverse proteins in a temporal frame would reflect critical responses to EMD *in vivo*. Some regenerative actions of amelogenin and ameloblastin are replicated in EMD.

EMD enhances yields of 5α-dihydrotestosterone (DHT), a marker of oxidative stress and wound healing in both MG63 osteoblasts and human periosteal fibroblasts *in vitro*. There were elevated yields of DHT in response to EMD, both alone and in combination with glutathione; to overcome the oxidative effects of nicotine in the culture [21]. The direct actions of DHT on matrix synthesis and oxidative stress, confirm that EMD has scope for applications in bone regeneration and tissue engineering. The anabolic potential of a deproteinised natural cancellous bone mineral was validated in culture, in order to establish its proanabolic actions in human periosteal fibroblasts *in vitro* [22]. Enzyme assays were performed for the biologically active androgen 5α-dihydrotestosterone (DHT) as a marker of wound repair, in the presence of minocycline, alone and in combination with the bone mineral. Minocycline was used as a standard for confirmation of responses to bone mineral, in view of documentation in the literature of its proanabolic effects. These findings reinforce the proanabolic actions of deproteinised bone mineral on periosteal fibroblasts with applications for bone regeneration and tissue engineering.

Excessive tooth mobility and smoking could have a negative influence on periodontal regeneration. It is recommended that early regenerative therapy of intrabony defects offers good potential for periodontal regeneration over open flap debridement alone, with due consideration of case selection, defect morphology, principles of regenerative biology and potential adverse modifying factors. Treatment should be followed by an effective maintenance programme for long-term sustenance. These findings have been confirmed in a systematic review [23], paying attention to patient-, tooth-, site- and procedural considerations. Long-term studies indicate that improved clinical parameters can be maintained for a period of 10 years, even amongst teeth that are severely compromised, indicative of a favourable long-term prognosis.

Preclinical histological studies have evaluated the regenerative efficacy of biomaterials alone or in combination for the treatment of periodontal intrabony defects, using systematic review methods [24]. New periodontal ligament, cementum and bone parameters were assessed in a linear manner in relation to proportions of root length. Barrier membranes, grafting materials and growth factors/proteins were evaluated for the management of intrabony defects after a healing period of at least 6 weeks. Heterogeneity of data precluded a meta-analysis. Flap surgery in conjunction with biomaterials in various combinations showed the best results for periodontal regeneration in comparison with flap surgery alone. Autografts demonstrated the most favourable outcome amongst the biomaterials evaluated.

The efficacy of enamel matrix derivative as an effective biological agent for periodontal regeneration has been shown in histological and controlled clinical studies, with substantial improvement in clinical parameters. The effects of EMD alone, compared with its combined applications with diverse bone grafting materials have been reviewed [25]. It demonstrates that EMD in combination with some bone grafts enhances the regeneration of periodontal defects involving furcations and intrabony sites. However there is some variation in the results of studies conducted and further controlled clinical trials are required.

Low power GaAlAs (gallium-aluminium-arsenide) laser treatment was shown to have a positive impact on periodontal wound healing in conjunction with placement of bioactive glass in wounds created in rat mandibles [26]; and in human infrabony defects using a split-mouth design [27]. There was significant bone infill at defect sites demonstrated by histopathology and radiology. Replication of lost tissues of the periodontium is a challenging goal. Using combined therapy for bone and tissue regeneration with bioactive adjuncts, results in significantly less variation in treatment outcome; than using surgical flap procedures alone in the absence of adjunctive agents.

The effects of autologous platelet concentrate alone or in combination with other materials in the management of intrabony defects, have been evaluated in a systematic review of Medline and the Cochrane Central Register of Controlled Trials; using clinical and radiographic periodontal outcome measures demonstrating a follow-up period of at least 9 months [28]. Open flap debridement was compared with additional defect grafts, using autogenous bone or bone substitutes, in the presence or absence of a covering membrane for guided tissue regeneration (GTR). The periodontal parameters tested showed significant additive effects in response to platelet rich fibrin when used with open flap debridement. Platelet rich plasma shows significant enhancement in conjunction with bone grafts, while it was not effective with GTR procedures. Further work is required to clarify the applications of other forms of autologous platelet concentrate.

Periodontal regenerative potential and *in vivo* biocompatibility of enzymatically solidified chitosan hydrogels, with or without periodontal ligament cells have been evaluated in rat intra-bony defects [29]. Untreated defects were used as controls.

Periodontal ligament cells remained viable when contained in chitosan hydrogels prior to transplantation; the gel was degraded 4 weeks after implantation, with no adverse effects on tissues. No cell signals were detected in the cell-impregnated gels 4 weeks after transplantation, making it difficult to ascertain the effect of impregnated cells. However, the hydrogels are biocompatible and biodegradable. Even in the absence of cells they improve parameters of periodontal wound healing, comprising alveolar bone and a functional periodontal ligament. Further work is required on their applications as carriers of cells.

Enzymatic control over the gelation of chitosan-based hydrogels for the delivery of periodontal ligament cells has been studied [30]. Results indicate that variation of urea and urease concentrations could control the gelation time, strength and degradation rate of chitosan gels. Periodontal ligament cells could remain viable within the hydrogels for 30 days. On degradation of the hydrogel, cells released at 3, 15 and 30 days are capable of colony formation and osteogenic differentiation. Enzymatic control over the gelation of chitosan hydrogels, provides means of delivering periodontal ligament cells effectively, at the required site.

Periodontal regenerative capacity, is seen in periodontal ligament cells (PDLC) positive for the stromal cell antigen STRO-1 and in unsorted PDLCs. Differences between the unsorted PDLCs and expanded STRO-1 cells have not been reported previously. In view of the influence of Wnt3a on cell proliferation, it could benefit expansion of PDLC. These interactions prompted a study to evaluate the behavior of PDLCs in response to Wnt3a and STRO-1 cell sorting [31]; hPDLC were sorted for STRO-1 positive cells which were expanded and compared with unsorted parental cells. Subsequent exposure of cells to Wnt3a, enabled comparison for cell proliferation, renewal and osteogenic differentiation. There were no differences between STRO-1 sorted and unsorted parental cells with regard to cell proliferation and osteogenic capacity. There was significant enhancement of proliferation and self-renewal of hPDLCs in response to Wnt3a, demonstrated by an attenuated cell replication period, greater DNA content and enhanced expression of the self-renewal gene Oct4. These activities were promoted by Wnt3a over 5 passages without any change, in all cells; with no superior effects demonstrated by expanded STRO-1-sorted hPDLCs.

Management of Gingival Recession Defects

Root coverage of gingival recession defects is an important aspect of periodontal regeneration. A consensus report based on appraising a systematic review on the management of recession defects on single and multiple teeth; and relevant clinical debate emerged positive for consistent treatment outcome, especially when there was no interdental bone loss [32]. Sub-epithelial connective tissue grafts have shown the best results for root coverage. Alternatives to autogenous donor tissue are allogeneic dermal matrix grafts and enamel matrix derivative in conjunction with coronally advanced flap procedures. Multiple recession defects, recession at sites other than maxillary canines and premolars, site-specific and patient-reported factors for procedural outcome, require further scrutiny. Surgical interventions for the coverage of root surfaces have been evaluated for the strength of scientific evidence in order to recommend certain procedures [33]. Soft tissue deficiencies at implants, single and multiple recessions were assessed. There was a moderate strength of evidence to support the following concepts: The outcome of coronally advanced flaps is improved by the addition of connective tissue grafts. It is also improved by the addition of enamel matrix derivative (EMD). Treatment of multiple recession sites requires more care. It is possible to obtain complete root coverage with some interdental bone loss. Although several procedures are available for soft tissue coverage of implants, greater heterogeneity amongst studies done, makes it difficult to draw conclusions at the present time.

It is concluded by the group that periodontal plastic surgery is complex and technique sensitive, requiring advanced skills. Autologous connective tissue grafts or EMD in conjunction with coronally advanced flaps enhance complete root coverage, where single recessions at maxillary anterior and premolar teeth may be considered; requiring evaluation in the context of increased morbidity at the donor site. Further work needs to research alternatives to autologous grafting of soft tissues at single/multiple recession sites; and methods applicable to recession defects with interdental bone loss and soft tissue loss at implants.

A collagen matrix (CM) derived from porcine tissue is an alternative to palatal connective tissue grafts, to be used in conjunction with coronally advanced flaps for the management of Miller Class 1 and ll gingival recession defects [34]. However its efficacy as an alternative to connective tissue grafts

(CTG), at single or multiple recession sites is not known. The clinical outcome following treatment of Miller Class 1 and ll (no interdental bone loss) multiple, adjacent gingival recession cases, using a modified coronally advanced tunnel technique; in conjunction with CM or CTG has been evaluated in a split mouth study design. CM is effective in reducing surgical time and patient morbidity which makes it a potential alternative to CTG. However, there was reduced complete root coverage, over cases treated with connective tissue grafting, in conjunction with a modified coronally advanced tunnel technique; for Miller Class 1 and ll multiple adjacent gingival recession defects.

Regeneration of damaged organs or tissues is the ultimate outcome of treatment. Concepts of regenerative medicine and tissue engineering are used effectively for a range of applications. There are several options for harvesting and using adult somatic mesenchymal stem cells, including the oral cavity. They were originally thought to be restricted developmentally to specific cell lineages related to their tissue of origin. However it has been demonstrated that they have a wide differentiation potential, covering most tissues derived from mesenchyme. The potential for successful mesenchymal cell therapy in humans has been demonstrated in animal research. Isolation of cells from bone marrow is an invasive procedure which could be fraught with morbidity at the site and other complications; with the added disadvantage of low cell numbers, requiring *ex-vivo* expansion of cells. Adult autologous stem cells should ideally be relatively easy to obtain, with minimal patient morbidity; and available in relatively large numbers without the need for extensive cell expansion. In this regard, the oral cavity and gingivae in particular, provide exceptionally easy access for harvesting stem cells; with minimal morbidity at the site due to rapid healing capacity of gingivae. Tissue engineering has advanced over the years. However, cell based therapy is confined to clinical trials and not performed routinely. The preparation of biological products needs to be standardized, with suitable protocols and vehicles for cell transportation that are safe for patients; and the cells used, for the applications required. These requirements would need to be resolved satisfactorily prior to using stem cells as a therapeutic alternative.

Focused regeneration of periodontal tissue components is challenging, due to multiple isoforms associated with redundant molecules. They are capable of auto-induced bone formation driven by soluble osteogenic molecular signals. A diverse range of pleiotropic actions of soluble molecular signals in soft and hard tissue, regulate epithelial/mesenchymal tissue interactions. Their functional profile is of relevance in a clinical therapeutic context [35]. Fine tuning of seemingly redundant isoforms of human osteogenic proteins, would result in more focused targeted therapy for regenerative tissue engineering, with greater biological significance. Re-shaping and re-profiling multiple targets towards improved streamlined activity, assist accurate dissemination of active agents to matrix and bone. This is pivotal to regenerative procedures, for delivery of stimulatory agents over critical temporal phases of wound healing, using slow release devices, loaded scaffolds and vehicular microcapsules. Relevant techniques for tissue engineering and gene therapy, enhance protein expression and cell expansion. These concepts are reviewed.

There is a constant search for consistent, robust regenerative strategies, despite diverse methods and biomaterials that have enhanced tissue engineering technology; for improved healing potential in periodontal bone defects. They include regenerative surgical procedures, using a spectrum of biomimetics, growth factors and matrices. Replication of biologically effective functional tissue is an elusive goal. Regeneration of different components for functional stability has been achieved using a combination of bone replacement grafts and guided tissue/ bone regeneration. A spliced membrane is used in this technique to prevent epithelial ingress; thus encouraging regeneration of mesenchymal components in the wound-healing compartment, between the denuded root surface and supporting bone. The biological potential is enhanced by using growth-promoting agents [36]. There is significantly less variation in clinical periodontal attachment levels, when barrier membranes are combined with open flap debridement; compared with flap surgery alone. Grafting with demineralised bone matrix has shown more predictable bony infill than flap surgery alone. However, some variation in treatment outcome of infrabony defects using combined methods is expected. This is determined by variation in defect morphology, depth and severity of attachment loss at baseline; and operator sensitivity. Combined therapy could enhance predictability of outcome at sites that may not respond well to flap surgery alone.

Chapter 3

Biomarkers of Cell Differentiation and Growth Promoting Agents

Mesenchymal stem cells have good potential for trans-differentiation into a range of adult cell types including endothelial cells. Wharton's jelly obtained from foeto-placental tissue is a superior source of mesenchymal progenitor stem cells with low immunogenicity, suitable for enhancing tissue repair. Endothelial cells derived from human mesenchymal stem cells obtained from Wharton's jelly (hWMSCs) were evaluated in this context. Mesenchymal and endothelial markers were used for cell phenotyping following induction of endothelial trans-differentiation; demonstrated by their ability to synthesize nitric oxide and expression of endothelial markers [37]. Human WMScs could differentiate into adipocytes, osteocytes, chondrocytes and endothelial cells; they show low expression for endothelial markers prior to induction and high levels of mesenchymal markers. When compared with animals injected with undifferentiated hWMSCs, cells with endothelial differentiation accelerated wound healing in a mouse model of skin injury. Similar effects are seen in animals injected with conditioned media from endothelial differentiation cultures. This study defines potential for endothelial trans-differentiation of hWMSCs. These differentiated endothelial cells could produce soluble pro-angiogenic factors and enhance tissue repair by promoting neovascularization.

In view of limited potential for repair of damaged cartilage, autologous chondrocyte implantation is an effective option, although there would be an element of donor site morbidity; minimized by harvesting autologous mesenchymal stem cells cultured from chondrocytes. The umbilical cord, an ecto-embryologic tissue is a good source of cells in abundance, readily isolated. It is accessible and painless for harvesting cells, with no ethical issues. Human WMScs cultured in high density show positive protein expression of CD90, c-kit, Sca1, SH2 and SH3, indicative of mesenchymal differentiation seen in bone marrow stomal cells; as well as expression of the chondrocyte markers Sox-9 and Col-2A1. Extracellular cartilage matrix secretion is seen, when high density hWMSCs are cultured with TGFβ1 and dexamethasone. It is integrated in a thin layer of cell-based membrane [38]. In a rotary cell culture system it forms an opaque cartilage-like tissue, larger and denser than when conventional pellet culture is used. At 3 weeks in culture, glycosaminoglycan and type ll collagen content increased significantly. Low immunogenicity and lack of haematopoietic cells in Wharton's jelly enable samples of greater purity. It has potential for constructing tissue-engineered cartilage.

Bone metabolism is regulated by osteocytes derived from osteoblasts which communicate with other cells of a similar lineage. The mature osteocyte expresses the protein sclerostin, which has inverse effects on bone mass, being a negative regulator. In physiological conditions, sclerostin acts on osteoblasts at the bone interphase and shows differential expression in response to inflammatory triggers, mechanical loading and hormones such as PTH and oestrogen. Dysregulation of sclerostin has been seen in pathologies such as osteoporosis-related fractures, failed osseointegration of implants and genetically modulated diseases affecting bone mass [39]. Phase lll clinical trials are currently in progress working on an antibody that targets sclerostin. It reduces endogenous levels of sclerostin and increases bone mineral density. The osteocyte is an indispensable, versatile bone cell. Its location within bone, communication with the systemic circulation and other cells of a similar lineage; could provide opportunities for the management of a range of conditions in the field of orthopaedics. An extensive dendritic network helps the process.

Due to the specialized morphology and molecular signature of osteocytes trapped within newly mineralized bone matrix, they have a unique cellular identity. These characteristics allow them to function as bone response modulators in their microenvironment, in response to mechanical stress [40]. Sclerostin, a key molecule in mechano-transduction, is produced by osteocytes. Its expression is suppressed by mechanical loading and induced on removal of the load. Its role as an important mediator of the remodelling apparatus, by unifying mechanical, local and hormonal signals recognized by osteocytes, is reviewed. There is interplay beween mechanical loading and low sclerostin levels, associated with activation of Wnt-canonical signalling and bone formation. Lack of loading induces high sclerostin levels leading to bone resorption initiated by osteoblasts and osteoclasts, via suppression of Wnt-canonical-β-catenin signalling. This results in Wnt-noncanonical and/other pathways in these cells, leading to bone resorption. Altered sclerostin levels regulate diffential production of RANKL and OPG, creating a dynamic duo, resulting in bone remodelling with either resorption or bone formation. There are other mechanisms which affect mineralization of formed matrices. These opposing regulatory phases result in adaptive bone remodelling, with osteocytes functioning as a discrete unit. The osteocyte network plays a central role in regulating bone responses to mechanical loading or the lack of loading, leading to bone formation or resorption respectively.

Osteocytes play a significant role in responding to hormonal and mechanical stimuli for the coordinated functions of osteoblasts and osteoclasts. Sclerostin inhibits bone formation and in bone, it is primarily expressed in osteocytes. Down-regulation of sclerostin by anabolic stimuli indicates a mechanism whereby osteocytes affect osteoblast metabolism. Osteocytes are actively engaged in recruitment of osteoclasts and bone remodelling. Apoptotic osteocytes trigger signals which have not been identified. They are able to attract osteoclast precursors to sites of remodelling where they differentiate into mature bone-resorbing osteoclasts [41]. Osteocytes also generate the molecules OPG (osteoprotegerin) and RANK (receptor activator of nuclear factor-kappa B), that regulate osteoclasts and their activity. Bone resorption is markedly affected by genetic manipulation of either of these molecules in the mouse genome, due to their altered genetic expression. The novel concept of osteocyte-driven bone remodelling, influences our understanding of current therapies, which contribute to bone resorption and formation.

The CCN family of proteins (an acronym derived from the first 3 members of the family that were discovered) is a group of matricellular proteins including connective tissue growth factor (CTGF). It was discovered rather early and is also known as CCN2. This unique signalling modulator has novel molecular properties and actions. Due to its interactions with multiple molecules, diverse context-specific biological outcomes are seen, dependent on the microenvironment [42]. CCN2 conducts coordinated development of several tissues including cartilage and bone, by regulating extracellular signalling molecules and acting as a hub via a molecular network. Its physiological and pathological roles which include excessive fibrosis and malignant changes in organs and tissues are reviewed.

Mesenchymal stem cells (MSCs) are effective progenitor cells that are capable of repair and regeneration of impaired tissue. The effect of pre-treatment of MSCs with isosorbide dinitrate (ISDN) an organic nitrate, in attenuating effects of their senescence has been studied. Senescence was induced in MSCs by treating them with high concentrations of glucose. It was markedly reduced in cells that were pre-treated with ISDN [43]. This was indicated by senescence-associated biomarkers such as p21 expression, mRNA levels of DNA methytransferase 1 (DNMT1), senescence-associated galactosidase (SA-β-gal) activity and embryo chondrocyte expressed gene1 (DEC1). It is relevant that glucose-induced senescent MSCs showed marked down-regulation of ERK activity and forkhead box M1 (FOXM1) expression, which ISDN preconditioning is able to reverse. Inhibition of ERK phosphorylation and downregulation of FOXM1 abolished the beneficial effects of ISDN. Amongst the senescence-associated miR-130 family, miR-130b mediates beneficial effects of ISDN. It is relevant that knockout of miR-130b, significantly reverses the beneficial effects of ISDN against senescence of MSCs. In addition, downregulation of ERK phosphorylation or FOXm1 expression decreased the expression level of miR-130b. The favourable effects of ISDN, against high glucose-induced MSC senescence, mediated via the activation of ERK/FOXM1 pathway; and the up-regulation of miR-130b have been demonstrated for the first time.

Other growth promoting agents are addressed in Chapter 2 under periodontal regeneration, linked to relevant subject areas and also covered in other chapters.

Chapter 4

Periosteal Cell Sheets and Tissue Matrix

The regenerative potential of periosteum is underestimated in Dentistry, in the context of tissue regeneration of lost tissue. The extent of utilization of autogenous periosteum does not compare with that in Medicine [44]. Periosteum could be considered to be a bone envelope of osteoprogenitor cells with tremendous regenerative potential, rich in fibroblasts, osteoblasts and stem cell progenitors; with the ability to differentiate into multiple mesenchymal cell lineages. It is a rich source of cells for bone tissue engineering, readily harvested from the oral cavity. It functions as an appropriate reservoir of progenitor cells in response to stimuli, with a rapid turnover. Periosteal cells are an effective source of tissue regeneration and restoration, including cementum and periodontal ligament; while periosteal cell sheets constitute effective material for grafting. The development of biomimetic tissue-engineered periosteum for replacement or enhancement could be optimized, with improved knowledge of its smart material characteristics; for a wider scope of applications in regenerative Medicine [45] and Dentistry. These applications demonstrate the role of microRNAs in modulating gene expression, mature strand sequences that function optimally in microRNAs that do not occur naturally, differentiation of osteoblasts and tissue repair [46]; used in conjunction with constructs for mimicry of ECM. There is potential for utilizing periosteum as a smart biomaterial, with prior knowledge of the immune privilege of progenitor cells derived from periosteum.

The development of an engineered periosteum is a significant step towards bone regenerative therapy, as a functional periosteum would accelerate bone formation. It is possible to generate cell sheets from bone marrow stromal cells in order to regenerate periosteum. Sheets of bone marrow stromal cells wrapped around calcium phosphate scaffolds and implanted in mice, produced a functional periosteum-like tissue, confirmed by tissue morphology and protein expression. Other studies report engineering of periosteum, by combining stromal cells with collagen gel scaffolding or using stromal cell sheets. These studies focused on bone regeneration rather than characterization of a functional periosteum. Although bone formation is essential, this model identifies continued radial bone growth in physiological conditions. TGF-β1 has been shown to enhance the formation of periosteum, by increasing its cellularity and providing more progenitor cells in bone defects. Periosteal grafts pre-treated with TGF-β1 resulted in increased periosteal thickness [47]; TGF-β1 also enhances the expression of periostin. The addition of TGF-β1 to the bone marrow stromal cell sheets prior to their placement around calcium phosphate pellets could enhance periosteal regeneration in this construct. The regeneration of periosteum in this model demonstrates a promising technique for periosteal engineering and cell delivery for bone regenerative therapies. Autologous cell sheets are readily translated for clinical applications without the need for exogenous materials; larger scale studies on periosteal engineering systems could promote their usage.

It has been demonstrated that multilayered periosteal sheets prepared from explants of alveolar periosteum, have applications for periodontal regeneration with effective osteogenic potential. Stem cell culture media (MesenPRO) have been used to develop more potent expanded periosteal cell sheets [48]. Significantly stronger osteogenic potential was demonstrated *in vivo* when these cell sheets were implanted in nude mice; and Mesen PRO enhanced the formation of thicker multilayers of cells *in vitro*. CD146 positive cells were notably increased, a significant finding in view of the fact that CD146 is a marker for osteogenic progenitor cells found in the stroma of bone marrow. Induction of CD146-positive cells by Mesen PRO in periosteal cell sheets has notable applications for enhancing osteogenesis in clinical regenerative procedures.

A functional periosteum provides progenitor cells, for acceleration of healing in bone defects, by supplying an effective source of appropriate cells. The hypothesis that bone marrow stromal cells (BMSCs) could be used to engineer functional periosteal tissues has been studied. BMSCs were cultured to hyperconfluence, aiding the production of sufficient extrcellular matrix in substantial cell sheets. Subcutaneous implantation of calcium phosphate pellets wrapped in these cell sheets was compared for histological parameters, with implantation of pellets in the absence of cell sheets, over an 8 week period [49]. The formation of bone and periosteum were analysed using tissue morphology and the expression of tissue-specific protein. It is significant that pellets wrapped in cell sheets produce bone-like tissue on the calcium phosphate scaffolds; encased in a periosteum-like tissue which was characterized for the expression of periostin and morphological parameters. The implanted pellets alone did not produce bone. These findings indicate that sheet technology could contribute to regeneration of a functional periosteum with applications in bone surgery.

Periostin, an extracellular matrix protein expressed by periosteal osteoblasts and preosteoblasts, also known as osteoblast-specific factor-2, functions as a cell adhesion molecule. Periostin is found in a relatively small number of tissues in the body and significantly not expressed in bone matrix or endosteum, which makes it a periosteum-specific marker. Cell sheet technology has numerous applications in regenerative therapies such as organ tissue repair and corneal regeneration. This method involves matrix induction in hyperconfluent cultured cells for the purpose of fabricating a robust, functional cell sheet. The prepared cell sheets could either be peeled with forceps or released from the dish if cultured on a suitable thermo-responsive polymer such as poly(N-isopropylacrylamide). As the periosteum is a sheet of tissue surrounding bone, its inclusion in a bone defect or regenerative scaffold would provide an avenue for periosteal engineering. Studies have demonstrated encouraging results for bone regeneration, using cell sheet technology; however, the development of a functional periosteum requires further molecular and structural characterization.

The anti-epileptic drug phenytoin modulates inflammatory wound healing by enhancing matrix synthesis and impairing its breakdown. It mimics an over-exuberant wound healing response. Several formulations of topical phenytoin have been used to promote wound healing, including a mucoadhesive phenytoin paste that demonstrates accelerated wound healing with reduced pain [50]. The metabolic responses of human periosteal fibroblasts *in vitro* were studied in response to phenytoin and histamine, simulating an inflammatory environment. In view of the antioxidant and matrix stimulatory actions of DHT (5α-dihydrotestosterone), it was used as the biomarker of inflammatory wound repair, using 14C-testosterone and 14C-4-androstenedione as independent substrates [51]. There were significant increases in yields of DHT in response to phenytoin and histamine using both substrates, indicative of their anabolic potential in periosteal fibroblasts. These findings hold promise for diverse applications of periosteal fibroblasts, in tissue repair and regeneration, in an inflammatory environment. Patents relevant to matrix synthesis are addressed in this context and its modulation by microRNAs, in an environment of inflammatory healing.

Remarkable regenerative capacity of periosteum-derived cells and their applications in tissue engineering and translational therapies, drive further elucidation of their role in this context. Their unique features make them ideal candidates for translational research and clinical applications, comparable to those of bone marrow stromal cells [52]. Some of these characteristics include differentiation and tissue growth enhancing properties. These considerations open pathways for banking periosteum-derived cells as progenitors, akin to cells derived from umbilical perinatal tissue sources. Clarification of similarity and diversity amongst multipotent cells from distinct tissue niches; and their capacity to differentiate and induce tissue regeneration, would improve their scope for translational applications in tissue engineering and regenerative Medicine/Dentistry. The entire population of osteoblasts at periosteal, endosteal and trabecular bone sites within bone marrow, has embryonic perichondrial origins [53]. Activation, expansion and differentiation of periosteal progenitor cells are considered to be pivotal as templates for neovacularisation, bone formation and remodelling that follow. The periosteum acts as a reservoir of molecules that modulate cell behavior, being a unique niche of pluripotent cells. It has advanced smart material characteristics regulated by its mechanical, chemical and biological status. Recognition of its inherent regenerative and tissue-building capacity paves the way for harnessing these properties more effectively.

The molecular and cellular mechanisms associated with the periosteal contribution to bone regeneration are increasingly recognized. Relative contributions of periosteum and endosteum to bone regeneration are better defined with lineage tracing analytical studies and those in knockout transgenic mice; including critical roles of BMP, FGF, PDGF, Wnt and cell signalling during inflammation. They influence periosteum-mediated bone regeneration for regenerative therapy, applicable to Medicine and Dentistry [54]. Some of these concepts have been addressed, in the context of harnessing periosteum for bone regenerative tissue engineering.

Chapter 5

Functions of Hydrogels in Tissue Regeneration

Tissue engineering has had tremendous impact on effective regenerative medicine, over the decades. Its clinical applications have been relatively limited due to restrictions on biomaterials that are approved for applications in humans. As a result, biodegradable polymers, approved over 30 years ago, are still in vogue for applications in humans. During normal development and morphogenesis of tissue, there is close interaction between cells and extracellular matrix. However, although simple polymers provide structural support for the development of new tissues, they may not mimic complex biological interactions between progenitor cells and matrices, required for functional tissue regeneration. Future advances in tissue engineering require smart biomaterials [55] for clinical translation, engaged in active functional tissue formation. Hydrogels mimic cell matrices closely and comprise natural or synthetic polymer systems which are able to absorb water. In view of their increasing applications in regenerative Medicine/Dentistry, several advances have been made in hydrogel chemistry; with improved control of cell fate and cell/tissue interactions, in a tissue environment of oxidative stress and inflammation. New understanding of these concepts and recent advances are reviewed [56].

Regenerative therapy has evolved over the years with several effective applications, where previous approaches may have failed. Semisynthetic extracellular matrix mimetic sECM, a. has the capacity to convey cells at the site of delivery and retain them; b. has biochemical properties that may be adapted to each tissue type, for optimal function. A simple design approach is utilized with a deconstructed minimalist sECM for customization *in situ* [57]. Semisynthetic ECM is an essential component for improved outcome in cell-based therapies, due to the critical role of ECM in tissue formation, maintenance, regulation and function. For successful delivery of progenitor/stem cells, clinically viable synthetic ECMs are crucial for therapeutic localization of delivered cells. They can be fine-tuned for specific progenitor cell types. Synthetic ECMs are available as porous solids, hydrogels or nanofibres (e.g electrospun). Hydrogels and nanofibres reproduce the 3D interactive environment of ECM, unlike porous, solid scaffolds which also promote transport, cell seeding, migration and integration with existing tissue; but are at best 2-dimensional with regard to cellular activity. Hydrogels have the benefit of cross-linking *in situ*, to allow cell infiltration for the creation of a 3D structure immediately. Coversely, it is not possible to form electrospun matrices with nanoscale pores *in situ*. This excludes the possibility of immediate cell movement into the matrix that is spun. Hydrogels have the flexibility and diversity of a superior class of compound and have the capacity to become optimized sECMs.

The thiol-norbornene (thiol-ene) photoclick hydrogels have diverse applications for tissue engineering. Their wide applications in tissue engineering and regenerative medicine have been reported in several laboratories. In addition to musculo-skeletal functions, these include valvular, vascular, stem cell culture applications, tissue engineering relevant to organ repair and differentiation capacity. Thiol-norbornene hydrogel cross-linking and degradation mechanisms, regulatory actions as well as their drug-delivery and tissue engineering applications, have been addressed in a review [58]. They are cross-linked through orthogonal reactions between multi-functional norbornene-modified macromers such as poly(ethylene glycol, hyaluronic acid, gelatin and sulfhydryl-containing linkers such as bis-cycteine peptides. Reactions are light-mediated with low levels of photoinitiator. The gelation of thiol-norbornene hydrogels does not need additional co-initiator or co-monomer, when long-wave UV light or visible light is used instead. Selection of materials controls cross-linking and degradation behavior of thiol-norbornene hydrogels. However, the biophysical and biochemical properties of the gels could be controlled independently, in view of orthogonal reactions between norbornene and thiol moieties. Lack of inhibition of the cross-linking step enhancement of thio-norbornene hydrogels by oxygen, incurs more rapid, significantly cytocompatible gelation; when compared with chain-growth polymerized hydrogels, under similar gelation conditions. These hydrogels have been prepared as substrates that can be fine-tuned for 2D cell culture, as scaffolds for 3D-cell culture; and as affinity-based or protease-sensitive microgels or bulk gels, for drug delivery.

Coordinated applications of cells and scaffolds in bone regenerative medicine provide a potential strategy for bone regenerative therapy. Hydrogels show tremendous applications as scaffolds in minimally invasive procedures. The two main categories of hydrogels include collagen and oligo(poly(ethylene glycol)fumarate (OPF) hydrogels, representing natural and synthetically formed hydrogels. Optimal cell-loading, pertaining to distribution of cells within the hydrogels has been assessed [59]. Bone marrow and adipose tissue-derived MSCs have been studied in 3 loading methods comprising homogeneous cell encapsulation, location of cells in a sandwich between 2 hydrogel cell layers and spheroid encapsulation of cell pellets, using collagen and OPF hydrogel systems. Cells cultured in collagen hydrogels showed greater proliferation and osteogenic differentiation than in OPF hydrogels; indicative of cell behaviour being influenced by the type of hydrogel used. Adipose tissue MSCs showed greater proliferation and osteogenic properties than bone marrow MSCs. However the three loading methods showed no differences in mineralization. This disproved the hypothesis that sandwich and spheroid pellet loading would increase osteogenic capacity, in comparison with homogenous cell encapsulation. It was concluded that the latter and spheroid cell pellet loading show promise for bone substitutes that can be injected, in minimally invasive surgical regenerative procedures.

Stem cells are the initiators of tissue/organ regeneration, due to their potential for multilineage differentiation and self renewal. They are isolated from several tissue sources. However, their numbers are limited for direct clinical use without the critical intermediate step of cell expansion *in vitro* [60]. Despite their ability to expand *in vitro*, stem cells lose their ability to proliferate during passaging. Maintaining this capacity is one of the challenges of stem cell-based research. The latest developments in the capacity for self-renewal of stem cells, using strategic biomaterials during *in vitro* expansion are reviewed. The focus for future studies in the applications of stem cells for tissue regeneration, is highlighted. Stem cell renewal and differentiation are critical characteristics for replenishment and functions of the stem cell population, affecting tissue homeostasis. There is a considerable amount of documentation of processes involved, in controlling the fate of stem cells. Using biomaterial strategies, for modifying the physical environment of cells responding to mechanical stimuli, with mechanotransduction, avoids the use of chemicals. The cells respond to a mechanical cue, causing alterations in cell spreading and changes in internal cellular functions; resulting in a chemical signal within the cell, leading to changes in gene expression. These changes could occur directly due to changes in the cytoskeleton of the cell or indirectly via cascades of biochemical signalling [61]. These aspects of cell differentiation and renewal are addressed, in the context of the role of mechanotransduction and biomaterials that contribute to such changes.

With improved technology, new sophisticated biomaterials that induce spatial and temporal alterations of the cellular environment *in vitro,* are being created. The development of dynamic surfaces is an exciting step towards mimicking the changing chemistry and topography of the *in vivo* extracellular environment. By combining the concepts of chemical engineering, biomaterials that modulate substrate stiffness by altering pH or hydrogel composition have been produced [62, 63]. Thermally activated surfaces or oxidizable polymers could fine tune surface topography at sub-micrometre levels [64, 65]. Photo- or electrosensitive protecting groups are used to reveal cell adhesion ligands, that change the surface chemistry of biomaterials [66, 67, 68]. A cleavable linker in the system helps to release cell adhesion ligands [69, 70]. These techniques enable the generation of suitable cues on a temporal gradient, enabling stem cells to be studied in a dynamic *in vitro* environment, for comparison with an *in vivo* setting.

New, exciting avenues are available for the applications of stem cell therapy in regenerative Medicine and Dentistry, as increasing documentation clarifies their potential. The novel use of biomaterials could enhance applications of stem cells in regenerative biology, by providing *in vitro* mechanotransduction, without resorting to complex chemical cocktails of soluble factors, to mediate differentiation and cell growth. A better understanding of MSC adhesion/differentiation mechanisms has evolved, using nanoscale topography, regulation of stiffness and surface chemistry. The evolution of dynamic surfaces with the ability to switch on stem cell functions as required, enables replication of *in vivo* conditions within appropriate niches. These techniques are being developed with other types of stem cells, which would further enhance their applications in stem-cell regenerative therapies.

The discovery and applications of stem cells have provided an important driving force in the field of regenerative medicine. The impetus of MSCs, embryonic and induced pluripotent stem cells opens new avenues for tissue engineering; and potential for developing stem cell based therapies, for the management of diverse diseases [71]. Tissues with a range of cell lineages for derivation of multiple cell types could be produced from multipotent and pluripotent stem cells. A combined approach including bioreactors and biomimetic scaffolds provides an environment that is rich in stem cells; and representative of the microenvironment, for the generation of new tissue. Increased complexity in technology for development of bioactive scaffolds, reflects on their behaviour in modulating stem cell functions. Their composition comprising natural or synthetic materials, is formulated to drive cell regeneration and direct the fate of these cells. The cellular environment for tissue development requires critical conditions for these activities, such as growth factors and redox status, crucial for their regulated actions. Precise control of stem cell differentiation in culture would be an overarching goal of stem cell- based tissue engineering. Current developments in stem cell-based tissue engineering, utilizing several sources of stem cells and critical inducing agents have been reviewed. They comprise internal and external regulatory factors, affecting cell behaviour, mechanotransduction, biomaterials, growth factors and redox status.

Upregulation of downstream signalling targets of FAK such as JNK and ERK 1 / 2 are coordinated with raised Wnt signalling, demonstrated by microarray analysis and assays of pathway inhibition [72]. Elevated ALP activity and modulation of mineralized matrix formation, are sequenced by cyclical mechanical stretching. This induces the phosphorylation of FAK, enhanced expression and phosphorylation of Runx2, resulting in increased ALP activity [73]. Compressive or shear stress of fluids induces osteogenic differentiation of MSCs, involving a progressive cascade of responses, via several signalling pathways. Upregulation of osteogenesis-specific genes such as ALP, osteocalcin, Col 1 and osteopontin; and reorganization of the actin cytoskeleton as MSCs differentiate into osteoblasts, occur in response to signalling pathways such as MAPK, NO/cGMP/PKG and Ca2+signalling [74, 75, 76]. The combined effects of mechanical stretching and ECM composition in regulating the conversion of MSCs into an osteogenic lineage have been studied [73]. MSCs were cultured in basal medium, free of the influence of osteogenic supplements. They were subjected to mechanical stretching in a cyclical manner, on substrates coated with diverse ECM proteins such as type1 collagen, vitronectin, fibronectin and laminin. MSC differentiation into osteogenic phenotypes occurred in response to all ECM proteins studied. Phosphorylation of FAK, upregulated transcription, phosphorylation of RUNX2 and a resultant increase in ALP activity, leading to mineralized matrix deposition; were activated by the mechanical stretching cycles. It is relevant that fibronectin and laminin showed more significant results for stretch-induced osteogenic effects than either collagen type 1 or vitronectin.

Clarification of environmental cues that regulate appropriate cellular activity has resulted in advances in the field of tissue engineering. Diverse factors regulate proliferation and differentiation of stem cell progenitors into musculoskeletal lineages. The combined effects of multiple environmental cues would contribute to clinical applications of *in vitro* tissue engineering products. Considering studies of gingival fibroblasts, usually conducted under homoxic *in vitro* conditions, a hypoxic environment is more likely to represent *in vivo* conditions. It would also be relevant to identify environmental conditions that could improve the developing phenotypes of differentiated musculoskeletal cells. MSCs are capable of differentiating into osteoblasts quite readily *in vitro*; they would require physiologically engineered vascularised tissue that is functional in order to support osteogenic activity. For osteogenesis induced by embryonic stem cells, further work is required for regulating osteogenic lineage differentiation. However considerable progress has been made over the last decade towards creating *in vitro* engineered musculosleletal tissue for *in vivo* applications.

Cell-based therapy, including the treatment of musculoskeletal diseases is a critically important area of biomedical research. Both undifferentiated progenitor cells and differentiated cells have applications as initiators in this context. Using multipotent adult mesenchymal stem cells shows promise for therapeutic strategies. Cell delivery systems play a pivotal role in cell-based therapies, in addition to cell type. Cells could be delivered by direct injection or by grafting cell-seeded bioengineered constructs, derived from natural or synthetic biomaterials. This approach has the advantage of delivering a 3D construct, that would be compatible with mechanical properties of diverse musculoskeletal tissue; over direct injection of appropriate cells [77]. The applications for cell-based gene therapy and functional biomaterial scaffolds loaded with appropriate cells for tissue engineering and regeneration are reviewed.

Despite the cost of *ex vivo* culture of cells, there is good scope for cell delivery therapeutics for regenerative tissue engineering of the musculoskeletal system. Cells used with a biomaterial filler are pertinent for their applications in injured tissue, for chronic conditions such as rheumatoid arthritis and osteoarthritis, as documented. Cell-based therapies have shown efficacy in large scale human studies for broad clinical applications. For future use, which include matrix-based delivery of MSCs for bone and cartilage repair, cells show safety and effective results in phase 1 clinical trials. The utilization of factors that enhance certain types of repair is beneficial to musculoskeletal regeneration. In view of safety concerns, cell-induced protein and gene delivery are not standard protocols, for the management of chronic inflammatory diseases that are not life-threatening; despite their success and efficacy, reported in early phase 1 and phase ll clinical trials. The application of cells via biomaterials without resorting to additional factors is an area that is likely to show progress. Bone repair is particularly reponsive to cell therapy. Considering the fact that most indications for bone repair / regeneration are not life-threatening, safety aspects would be a primary concern for such applications. Cell therapy is likely to evolve and play a significant role in orthopaedic applications.

Chapter 6

Regenerative Medicine, Cell Signalling and Gene Delivery

Gene delivery has been used as a promising strategy at cell and tissue levels, for applications in regenerative medicine, for the creation/restoration of normal function. *Ex vivo* and *in vivo* applications have demonstrated successful gene delivery [78]. The capacity for proliferation and differentiation confers excellent potential for *ex vivo* gene delivery on certain cells, for applications in regenerative medicine. Intensive study in this context has enabled multipotent and pluripotent cells to be used in this capacity. The concepts of gene delivery and its applications in tissue engineering and regenerative medicine are reviewed. The properties and functions of stem cells, provide the foundation for detailed consideration of stem cell germ lineage, for gene delivery.

Normal tissue development and homeostasis are governed by TGF-β superfamily ligands. Disease states often demonstrate dysfunction of these ligands. They are characterized by well-defined structural and functional features. Engineering of the TGF-β superfamily ligand for therapeutic applications, particularly in regenerative medicine and musculoskeletal disorders has been reviewed [79]. New ligands can be created by structural mutation of receptor binding epitopes; by interchanging epitopes between ligands, resulting in functional properties that are individual, utilised for clinical applications. The results of engineered TGF-β prototype superfamily ligands show great potential and considerable untapped applications along these lines. They hold promise for future strategies and development of new biological innovations.

Canonical Wnt signalling is one of the critical signalling mechanisms for tooth development. However its role in inducing cementogenesis and promoting rejuvenation of lost periodontal tissue, due to periodontal disease is less well-defined. The role of canonical Wnt signal enhancing agents, on the differentiation of human periodontal ligament cementogenic cells *in vitro* and cementum repair; has been studied in a rat periodontal defect model [80]. Induction of canonical Wnt signalling was performed by injecting lithium chloride, sclerostin antibody and a lentiviral construct overexpressing β-catenin, locally. There was significant deposition of new cellular cementum and formation of a well orientated periodontal ligament, in response to activation of canonical Wnt signalling locally. These features were absent in the control group. The activators of the Wnt signalling pathway induced a significant increase in mineralization and alkaline phosphatase activity. There was expression of bone and cementum biomarkers: osteocalcin, osteopontin, cementum protein 1 and cementum attachment protein, in human periodontal ligament cells *in vitro*. These findings demonstrate that activation of the canonical Wnt signalling pathway could initiate cementum regeneration *in vivo;* and differentiation of human periodontal ligament cells into cementoblasts *in vitro*.

Due to certain inherent characteristics of gelatin such as ease of fabrication, electrostatic binding properties and proteolytic degradation characteristics, it has been used extensively as a popular vehicle for delivering a range of biomolecules for applications in tissue engineering and regenerative medicine. Modified gelatin offers better control over cross-linking of hydrogels, in comparison with traditional methods for cross-linking such as glutaraldehyde or methacrylate. The physical properties and growth factor delivery of gelatin methacrylate microparticles, fabricated with a range of diverse cross-linking densities of 15-90%, have been examined [81]. The elastic moduli of microparticles with less methacrylation were diminished with larger mesh sizes, compared with glutaraldehyde microparticles. Enhanced methacrylation correlated with smaller mesh sizes and increased moduli of elasticity. There was an inverse relationship between degradation and the density of microparticle cross-linking. This demonstrates a rapid rate of degradation in the least cross-linked gelatin methacrylate microparticles, which was comparable to glutaraldehyde microparticles.

It is relevant that gelatin methacrylate microparticles with lower cross-linking densities absorbed 10-fold greater relative quantities of growth factor, when compared with conventional glutaraldehyde cross-linked microparticles; despite a greater magnitude of gelatin content in the latter. Reduced cross linking density also showed greater efficacy, with more complete release of BMP-4 (bone morphogenetic protein) and bFGF (basic fibroblast growth factor); and enhanced rate of release when treated with collagenase [81]. This demonstrates greater flexibility of gelatin methacrylate microparticles, in providing an effective platform for delivery of growth factors. They show greater capacity for relative binding and regulation of proteolytic degradation. These features enhance their potential as a controlled release system for the delivery of growth factors.

Release kinetics of BMP-2 has been studied in diverse scaffolds and quantified using targeted mass spectrometry for a period extending to 70 days. A low dose of 1μg rhBMP-2 was immobilized by 4 methods designed to alter function, on poly (l-lactide)-co-(e-caprolactone)[(poly (LLA-co-CL)] scaffolds developed recently. BPM-2 was either physiosorbed on unmodified scaffolds (PHY), physiosorbed on scaffolds modified with nanodiamond particles (nDP-PHY), covalently linked to nDPs, to modify the scaffolds (nDP-COV) or encapsulated in microspheres distributed on the scaffolds (MICS). There was an initial spurt of release from PHY, while there was a more gradual and sustained release from MICS. In contrast, nDP-PHY and nDP-COV scaffolds did not show significant release; while nDP-PHYscaffolds maintained bioactivity of BMP-2 [82]. In the MICS and nDP-PHY scaffold groups, human MSCs cultured *in vitro* showed upregulated BMP-2 and osteocalcin gene expression at weeks 1and 3. BMP-2 extracellular protein levels assessed by ELISA and mineralization, confirmed by Alizarin red were also found to be highest amongst these groups. There was early expression of collagen type1 alpha 2 in cells grown on the PHY scaffolds. However, the scaffold was unable to sustain rhBMP-2 release in order to express mineralization.

Using a rat mandible critical-sized defect model, at 4 weeks post-implantation, there was an increased rate of bone regeneration in the PHY, nDP-PHY and MICS groups demonstrated by results of micro-CT and Masson trichrome. Due to lack of consistency in osteogenic potential in both *in vitro* and *in vivo* conditions, PHY scaffolds may not be appropriate for clinical use [82]. In contrast, nDP-PHY and MICS groups demonstrated satisfactory induction of bone regeneration under both conditions, in response to continuous low doses of BMP-2. The nDP-PHY scaffolds used here in critical-sized bone defects for the first time, are effective when compared with growth factors adsorbed on polymer alone. Adverse systemic side effects are prevented by the short distance effect.

Tissue engineering bone strategies provide significant opportunities for critical sized bone defects, in view of the limitations of current treatment options. Reproducing signals associated with bone development and regeneration is dependent on regulation of spatiotemporal delivery of growth factors, small molecules, nucleic acids and drugs. Effective modulation of signals would result in an interface of bone growth and regeneration, with other connective tissue matrices. This aids vascularisation of bone that has been tissue engineered. Concepts of modern technologies, that create spatially controlled patterns of bioactive agents, on interactive surfaces for 3D material constructs, specific signal presentation and pattern of delivery of bioactive factors, are reviewed [83]; underderscoring their significance in tissue engineering. As techniques of spatial resolution are enhanced, there is improved speed of patterning of *in vitro* models, for understanding responses of cells to spatially regulated biofactor signal delivery. This would lead to enhanced potential, for defining strategies that direct the capacity of specific spatial arrangements, for driving bone regeneration *in vivo*.

Mechanical properties of the extracellular matrix and anisotropic morphology, are important considerations for bioengineering of tissue equivalents. Collagen fibrils have particularly well-defined orientation throughout tissues and organs. Soluble collagen monomers can be regulated with regard to their alignment, unlike native insoluble collagen fibres where such prospects would be limited. A counter-rotating cone extrusion technology, for engineering tubular collagen constructs which have a defined anisotropy has been documented [84]. By modulating the divergence of inner and outer cone rotational speeds, collagen fibrils from bovine skin are extruded with orientation of fibres and bundles in tubular form. Shear forces generated by a combination of the direction of flow and rotation of the cone drive these changes. Variation in cone speeds manifests differences in elasticity and toughness of the collagen constructs. Rotational extrusion is an enhancing technology, for the synthesis and regulation of the an(isotropic) structure of collagen constructs, for applications in tissue engineering and regenerative medicine.

Chapter 7

Biomechanics of Stem Cells and Their Applications

Mesenchymal stem cells are able to synthesize and secrete bioactive regenerative molecules. Their ubiquitous nature and cell-characteristics make them one the most promising contenders for therapeutic applications. Adipose tissue-derived stem cells are increasingly used for a range of applications in humans and animals; as freshly isolated cells of the stromal vascular fraction (SVF) or as cultured adipose-derived stem cells (ASCs). Characterisation of ASCs in diverse animal species for tissue engineering potential, gene expression, immunophenotype, proliferation and differentiation has been done, particularly in canine and equine ASCs compared with feline cells which have been less well researched. ASC therapy has been delivered via several companies and used universally in dogs, cats and horses; although some of this activity does not have control from regulatory bodies, in many countries. The characterization and clinical use of SVF and ASCs have been reviewed for the first time, in diseases occurring spontaneously in veterinary animals [85]. There is a relatively large number of studies, addressing the applications of ASCs in induced lesions; compared with a relatively small number of studies that address ASC therapy in naturally occurring diseases in cats, dogs and horses. Diverse cell populations are used, with lack of adequate controls. This makes it difficult to be conclusive about the effects of ASC therapy, requiring further controlled studies to establish potential applications for ASCs in veterinary medicine.

Therapeutic use of haematopoietic stem cells derived from bone marrow in the 1960s, has lead to increased interest, in the study of undifferentiated progenitor cells that proliferate and differentiate in several tissues. A range of stem cells with diverse potential can be characterized. Despite the applications of embryonic stem cells, adult stem cells provide greater sourcing with interesting clinical applications. Mesenchymal stem cells (MSCs) from bone marrow, adipose tissue or MSCs isolated from Wharton's jelly have potential diverse applications in regenerative medicine. They have the added advantage of being obtained readily with minimal ethical considerations [86]. Over the past decade, these multipotent cells have generated interest. They are capable of immunomodulatory activity and are not associated with allogeneic immune responses. These properties are of particular interest and relevance in the field of regenerative medicine. Diverse clinical applications in bone and cartilage biology, cardiology, stroke medicine, diabetes, ophthalmology and organ construction are currently explored.

Clinical applications of stem cells for cell therapy and regeneration of tissues and organs would remain a challenge. While adult MSCs in particular, pose exciting possibilities in regenerative medicine, there are several concerns that need to be solved; regarding the amalgamation of scientific knowledge and technical considerations for the innovation of appropriate strategies. They include the quality of cells, mechanical signals and their role in tissue repair, enhanced yield of differentiated stem cells and appreciation of their heterogeneity which would direct their applications. One would consider predictable reproduction of a standard product, technical aspects regarding scaffold definition, long-term stability and culture conditions of cells and the impact of biomaterials used. Biological tissue could be grafted directly, via direct implantation of cells and cell-/gene therapy. Teratogenic, immunogenic, religious and legal issues are considerations relevant to the transportation of cells/tissues for *in vivo* applications. Certain cell types are less immunogenic, such as umbilical cord cells. This is a distinct advantage. While current knowledge on cell/tissue engineering holds considerable promise for future applications, further long-term randomised controlled clinical studies would provide more answers; with regard to some of the issues that have been raised.

Human-induced pluripotent stem cells (iPSC) can be generated with patient-orientated specificity. A wide spectrum of cellular phenotypes provides an effective source of autologous cells. Enhanced cellular functions of iPSC-derived fibroblasts hold promise as a significant cell source for personalised regenerative therapy. Biotechnological advances that are able to reprogramme somatic cells into pluripotent cells provide exciting regenerative applications. Controlled regulation and differentiation into functional fibroblasts from iPSC provide effective replenishment of fibroblasts. There is interesting evidence of augmented cellular function amongst the iPSC- derived fibroblast lineage, with improved biological potency [87]. This would benefit the development of novel personalized applications for stem cell therapies in oral diseases. There are questions that need to be answered before these cells can be used for prescribed applications routinely; such as the differentiation pathway of iPSC-derived cells along lineages that are similar to their origin. They also need to be screened for safety of therapeutic applications, their ability to sustain an induced phenotype; and capacity for tissue engineered development of effective 3D models, for optimal function and therapeutic applications. Delivery and integration of iPSC-derived fibroblasts in host tissue would be a challenge for functionality, sustenance and efficacy. Their biological potency would need to be harnessed for specific regenerative applications.

A novel porous bilayered scaffold was developed for the purpose of regenerating an osteochondral defect. It completely integrated silk fibroin (SF) and silk-nano calcium phosphate (silk-nanoCaP) layers and achieved homogeneous porosity distribution. The calcium phosphate phase was retained only in the silk-nanoCaP layer. There was good adhesion and proliferation of rat bone marrow mesenchymal stromal cells cultured on the scaffolds [88]. In osteogenic conditions, the silk-nanoCaP layer showed increased levels of alkaline phosphatase, over the silk layer. There was firm integration of the scaffold in host tissue, in the rabbit critical size osteochondral defect; demonstrating glycosaminoglycan regeneration and collagen ll positive cartilage in the silk layer, shown by immunohistochemical analysis. *De novo* bone ingrowths and vessel formation were observed in the silk-nanoCaP layer. Results shown, demonstrate the efficacy of these bilayered scaffolds, for the purpose of osteochhondral defect regeneration; in critical sized defects, using rat bone marrow mesenchymal stromal cells.

A simulated approach is used to design a novel nanocomposite system. Mineralization of hydroxyapatite is driven by nanoclays modified with amino acids, mimicking biomineralization [89]. A platform for material design and selection of appropriate biomaterials used in tissue engineering and regenerative medicine, is provided by this computational study. A nanocaly-hydroxyapatite (HAP) hybrid was designed, using nanoclay modified with unnatural amino acids and mineralizing HAP in the nanoclay galleries, simulating bio-mineralization; for the study of interactions with MSCs. Unnatural amino acids either occur naturally or are chemically synthesized and are non-proteinogenic. Their functional versatility and seemingly endless structural diversity, hold promise for wider applications; as chiral (symmetrical) building blocks and molecular scaffolds, for the construction of combinatorial libraries. They comprise a large collection of chemicals where reagents are identified, enabling refinement and optimization of potentially useful lead molecules. The hybrid (in situ HAP clay) is utilized for the fabrication of polycaprolactone (PCL)/*in situ* HAP clay films and scaffolds for bone regeneration [90]. Interactions between MSCs and PCL/*in situ* HAP clay composites in the form of films and scaffolds were studied using cell culture assays.

Attachment of MSCs, formation of mineralized ECM on PCL/*in situ* HAP clay films and infiltration of MSCs to interior aspects of PCL/*in situ* HAP clay scaffolds, were demonstrated with SEM imaging. MSCs induced mineralization of ECM in the absence of osteogenic supplementary agents. Imaging of the mineralized ECM generated on PCL/*in situ* HAP clay films indicated a hierarchical progression typical of natural bone, showing collagen and mineral components. Observation of cellular events during two-stage seeding experiments on the films, demonstrated similar stages to those seen during bone formation *in vivo;* and significantly elevated nanomechanical properties such as elastic moduli. The scaffolds showed increased degradation. These results demonstrate that the PCL/*in situ* HAP clay composites, are viable biomaterials for bone tissue engineering.

Tissue engineering strategy provides means of repairing mandibular defects, which is a clinical challenge. A small animal model has been used to study the effects of adipose-derived stem cells (ASCs) and bone morphogenetic protein-2 in 3D scaffolds, on mandibular repair [91]. ASC osteogenesis was enhanced by down-regulation of noggin expression, using a lentiviral short hairpin RNA strategy [ASCc(Nog-)]. 3D porous scaffolds were used for fabrication of natural polysaccharides of chitosan (CH) and chondroitin sulphate (CS). Apatite coatings were used to modify them further for more effective cellular responses and enhanced delivery of BMP-2. Critical sized bone defects were used in a rat mandibular model to study the efficacy of 3D-apatite-coated CH/CS scaffolds, supplemented with BMP-2 and ASCs(nog-). There was significant induction of rat mandibular defect regeneration in response to scaffolds treated with ASCs(Nog-) and BMP-2 at 8 weeks. This was demonstrated by tomography, histology and immunochemistry, compared with groups treated with ASCs(Nog-) or BMP-2 alone.

These results are suggestive of the efficacy of a combinatorial strategy comprising ASCs(Nog-)+BMP-2, in a microenvironment of 3D apatite scaffolds, for significant induction of mandibular regeneration. This model could be extrapolated for tissue engineering applications in large bone defects.

The mechanism of action of platelet-derived growth factor receptor β (PDGFRβ) signalling, on MSC proliferation and differentiation has been evaluated [92]. The main contributor to MSC proliferation in response to PDGFRβ activation was PI3K/Akt signalling, with a negative feedback loop between the two. Adipocytic differentiation of MSCs was blocked, by activation of Erk in response to PDGFRβ signalling; by inhibiting expression pathways. These findings indicate that the opposing fate decisions of proliferation and differentiation, for self-renewal of MSCs, are regulated by PDGFRβ-induced Akt and Erk pathways. This has important implications on tissue regenerative applications.

Epiblast stem cells (EpiSCs) in mice and rats are primed pluripotent stem cells (PSCs). EpiSCs could be reprogrammed to resemble embryonic stem cells (rESCs) in response to LIF (leukaemia inhibitor factor) - STAT3 (signal transducer and activator of transcription 3) signalling. However, low programming efficacy limits potential applications of rESCs in the generation of chimeras. The transcription factor, signal transducer and activator of transcription 3 (STAT3) are encoded by the STAT3 gene in humans. The protein encoded by this gene is a member of the STAT protein family. Members of the STAT family are phosphorylated by receptor-associated kinases; and subsequently act as transcription activators by forming homo- or hetero-dimers that translocate to the cell nucleus. This protein is activated via phosphorylation of tyrosine 705, in response to a range of cytokines and growth factors. They consist of interferons, epidermal growth factor (EGF), interleukin (IL-)5, bone morphogenetic protein 2 (BMP-2) and IL-10, including the hormone leptin. A dramatic improvement in efficacy of conversion from primed to naive-like PSCs, via upregulation of E-cadherin in the presence of LIF (leukaemia inhibitory factor) has been reported [93]. Blocking nuclear localization of β-catenin (cadherin-associated protein) with small-molecule inhibitors elevates reprogramming efficacy of mouse EpiSCs significantly. Activation of Wnt/β-catenin signals has been considered to be desirable for the maintenance of naive PSCs. However, the role of inhibition of nuclear translocation of β-catenin, in enhancing conversion of mouse EpiScs to naive-like PSCs (rESCs), has been validated in this study. It provides a better understanding of gene regulatory circuits involved in pluripotency and reprogramming of PSCs.

Chapter 8

Smart Biomaterials and Scaffolds

A tissue engineering scaffold provides form, mechanical support, cell proliferation and differentiation of seeded cells, resulting in a cellular architecture for the construction of new tissue, *in vitro* or *in vivo*. The majority of degradable biomaterials consist of synthetic polyesters which include poly[L-lactic acid] (PLLA) and poly[L-glycolic acid] (PLGA); and natural biological polymers comprising alginate, chitosan, collagen and fibrin [94]. Potential shapes, porosities and architecture of biomaterials are available in abundance, due to a multitude of fabrication techniques that have been devised [95, 96]. For the engineering of hard tissues, composites of synthetic and natural polymers in the presence or absence of bioactive ceramics; such as glasses and hydroxyapatite, have the capacity to yield materials with a range of porosities and strengths, particularly suitable for this purpose [97]. It is increasingly evident that for most tissue engineering applications, biomaterial scaffolds require to act in a more permanent capacity, than providing a temporary architecture for a developing tissue construct.

With the convergence of molecular cell biology and biomaterial science, new applications evolve in regenerative medicine; for coordinated orchestration of cell differentiation, expansion and tissue morphogenesis. Interactive biology between diverse components, underpins effective delivery of the concepts of tissue engineering. Physiological loading of bone was simulated, using calcium phosphate scaffolds and a bioreactor, in order to study the molecular response of hMSCs to loading [98]. Some immediate/early response genes associated with transcriptional regulation, are activated by loading, leading to induction of a larger gene pool responsible for osteoblast proliferation and differentiation. This provides valuable insight into signal transduction regulation pathways and molecular events; influencing osteogenic differentiation of MSCs, in response to simulated, physiological /mechanical stimulation.

It is relevant that key interactions between new classes of biomaterials, ECM and host responses are evaluated, utilizing tools that assess biocompatibility of traditional biodegradable polymers; and interactive ECM, including collagen. There is tremendous biodiversity amongst materials used in regenerative medicine and tissue engineering. Innovative methods are used to mimic the structure and function of ECM. They need further exploration and expansion, for application in biological systems; using tools that enhance comprehensive evaluation of new biomaterials in their ambient environment. Progressive evolution of newer regenerative technologies in human clinical trials, would continue to adhere to fundamental principles of biological interaction and biocompatibility. Diverse methods have been used to create durable bone, using appropriate implants to replace damaged tissue. The design of suitable nanostructured biomimetic agents is a novel challenge in tissue engineering and regenerative medicine. Electrospinning methods have been used to formulate non-woven scaffolds that mimic the fibrillar organization of extracellular bone matrix. The synthesis of a 3D, biomimetic, thick nanofibrous scaffold has been proposed, for the induction of bone regeneration [99]. It is formed by electrospinning biodegradable, bioresorbable poly (ε-caprolactone), which results in a scaffold of 1cm thickness, approved by the FDA. This scaffold was found to be an effective inducer of *in vivo* bone formation.

Thick electrospun biomimetic scaffolds would pose a problem for effective cell invasion. One could overcome this problem by using constructs of a desirable thickness and biomaterial properties such as porous electrospun meshes and self-assembling tissue spheroids which function in the capacity of building blocks. They are capable of tissue fusion, without the need for cell invasion. Pre-stretched electrospun meshes are able to support tissue spheroids without significant deformation; and are able to remain taut in cell culture. It was hypothesized that electospun scaffolds act as templates for support in a temporal manner, for rapid assembly of cell spheroids into upscale tissue components, such as tissue engineered vasculature. The potential for interference with the tissue fusion process when tissue spheroids are attached to pre-stretched polyurethane scaffolds has been studied [100]. Tissue spheroids are able to form tissue constructs on pre-stretched polyurethane electrospun matrices by a process of attachment, spreading and fusion, with some resultant hole-defects. Fibrogenic tissue growth factor-β is effective in inducing increased periostin and collagen synthesis, resulting in a dramatic reduction in the number and size of holes formed. It is relevant that when tissue spheroids fuse on a non-adhesive hydrogel, continuous tissue constructs are formed in the absence of holes, as shown in controls. In view of the findings demonstrating modulation of this process with suitable agents, a thin pre-stretched polyurethane electrospun scaffold, could serve as a template that supports biofabrication of thick tissue engineered constructs, overcoming the need for cell invasion; by using tissue spheroids in this application.

Considering their versatile biocompatibility, bioactivity, mechanical and degradation kinetics that can be modified, naturally derived polymeric biomaterials are used widely in tissue engineering. Materials with a range of applications are collagens, elastins, alginates, fibrins and silks. The advantages of using natural biopolymers for biomedical applications are their relative safety. They are processed using water-based environmentally friendly methods; and do not release cytotoxic degradation products. In view of these applications, natural biopolymers are used as scaffolds for tissue support and as matrices for the delivery of cells, for *in vivo* investigations. There is FDI approval of a range of novel biomaterials for clinical applications [101]. Delivery of oxygen and nutrition throughout the bulk of the engineered tissue, integration and vascularization of scaffolds on implantation within host tissue; are some of the limitations of enabling scaffolds, to support tissue engineering in large critically-sized defects. A porous scaffold platform formulated from biodegradable silk protein, containing a network of mimetic vasculature-like structure permeating the bulk of the scaffold; has been reported previously, to address these limitations. *In vivo* host tissue vascularization and integration are enhanced by utilizing hollow channels which are critical for cell infiltration and the delivery of nutrients and oxygen to the body of the scaffold [102]. Unique features of this protein biomaterial system comprising silk-based scaffolds, vascular structures and regulatory biomaterials, render this scaffold a robust model for applications in tissue engineering and regenerative medicine; underscored by its versatility for modulation of diseases.

Vascularisation of large 3D synthetic grafts remains a major challenge for tissue regenerative procedures. An electrochemical approach for detachment of cells (cell electrochemical detachment: CED) in order to form an integral endothelium has been employed. This has potential for prevascularisation of a collagen β-tricalcium phosphate (β-TCP) graft. Electrochemical detachment of an integral endothelium from a gold-plated glass rod, to a collagen-infiltrated, channelled β-TCP scaffold with micropores; results in an endothelium-lined microchannel containing the graft, when the glass rod is removed [103].

Robust endothelial microvascular formation and pre-vascularisation of the entire collagen/β-TCP integrated graft was demonstrated in perfusion cultures *in vivo*. There is evidence of established vascularization with a functional circulation, from the endothelium-lined microchannels within a relatively short period of time, with further temporal expansion. This is shown in subcutaneous implantation studies *in vivo*. The vasculature was also shown to invade prevascularised collagen / β-TCP grafts. The host vasculature demonstrated anastamoses with the preformed microvascular networks in the grafts. There is less vascular integration and anastamoses in collagen in the absence of support from rigid ceramic scaffolds. These concepts have potential, as an effective method of vascularising large grafts that are tissue engineered; by integrating CED-engineered, hydrogel-based, endothelium-lined microchannels with rigid channelled microporous scaffolds.

Repair and regeneration of large bone defects caused by trauma and disease are a major challenge primarily due to inadequate vascularisation. Superior biocompatibility and osteoconductivity of synthetic calcium phosphate (CaP) bioceramics, have enabled extensive applications as alternatives to autografts and allografts, in bone repair and regeneration. Effective vascularisation of large bone grafts is pivotal for their survival and enhanced integration within host tissue [104, 105]. Application of angiogenic growth factors could improve this process and enhance sustenance [106, 107], along with other strategies such as: endothelial cell monocultures/co-cultures with bone progenitor cells on scaffolds [108]; and insertion of bundles of vasculature in scaffolds [109]. However prevascularising grafts is a complex strategy and additional surgical measures may be required to assemble prefabricated vascular bundles [107].

As an alternative to the above strategy, the formation of microchannels in hydrogel-based matrices has been considered for simulation of vessels, to promote prevascularisation. The microchannels simulating vessels could enhance vascularisation, perfusion and carriage of essential nutrition and oxygen in a large graft [110]. Microchannels have been fabricated, using a variety of techniques such as layered assembly, 3D moulding [111], bioprinting [112] and photolithography [113, 114]. The technique involves perfusion of hollow channels created in the hydrogel with endothelial cells. Reorganization of the endothelial cells on the inner surfaces of channels results in the formation of endothelium [115, 116]. Integration of the formed microchannels with a rigid porous scaffold is one of the challenges in regenerative medicine and tissue engineering [111].

Intact endothelium has been engineered in collagen hydrogel, using an electrochemical cell detachment (CED) technique [117]. Human umbilical vein endothelial cells (HUVECc) cultured on an oligopeptide-coated glass rod until confluence is reached, acquire a surrounding casting of collagen hydrogel in a customized chamber. Subsequent detachment of the cells from the glass rod onto the surrounding collagen hydrogel, using the CED method results in a 'vascular endothelium' lining the microchannels [116, 117]. The driver in the CED technique is the sensitivity of the gold-complexed oligopeptide to electrical potentials [116], which cleaves chemical bonding between the gold-coated glass surface and the oligopeptide. This results in detachment of the intact endothelial cell layer and its adherence to the surrounding hydrogel. It leads to the formation of vascular microchannels for integration with scaffolds. The CED electrochemical approach for engineering endothelium is used to prevascularise collagen-β-tricalcium phosphate (β-TCP) grafts [103]. Its applications in fabricating endothelium-lined channels in microporous β-TCP scaffolds infiltrated with collagen, prompt progressive prevascularisation of the scaffold *in vitro* for graft expansion *in vivo*. This would establish cohesive vascularisation *in vivo*.

Regenerative therapies are now more consistent for regular applications in the reconstruction of cranio-maxillofacial defects. Effective vascularisation is key to the success of these therapeutic approaches. Extrinsic vascularisation may not always cater for the perfusion needs and complexities of craniofacial defects. An intrinsic axial vascularisation method using the arteriovenous loop has been addressed for bone regeneration in the mandible [118], in a systematic review of craniofacial tissue engineering. The versatility of the technique, challenges it poses and a protocol for the first clinical trial along these lines for mandibular reconstruction are discussed.

Chapter 9

The Role of MicroRNAs in Tissue Engineering

It has been shown in recent documentation that the small non-coding highly conserved microRNAs (miRNAs) are involved in diverse biological and pathological processes. Their main role is the regulation of post-transcriptional gene expression which leads to mRNA degradation and attenuation/activation of gene translational cues, by binding to their target mRNAs. These molecules serve as diagnostic biomarkers and have potential for targeting therapeutic applications for diverse conditions. Critical roles of miRNAs in different stages of diabetic wound healing and complications of DM are reviewed [119]. The expression of diverse miRNAs in fibroblasts is controlled by cytokines [120], of which, miR-155 is an example. Its transfection in a pulmonary fibrosis mouse model increases fibroblast migration leading to pulmonary fibrosis. A significantly reduced expression of miR-155 in mononuclear cells of Type 2 DM subjects has been shown [121]. This has also been demonstrated in diabetic mice; and the prevention of cardiac fibrosis when it is over-expressed in these mice [122]. The miRNA signature in diabetic wound healing has been analysed showing 14 miRNAs that are differentially expressed in diabetic skin [123]. Amongst these miRNAs, there is increased expression of miR-21 in diabetic skin which decreases during diabetic wound healing. There is dysregulation of diverse miRNAs involved in angiogenesis in diabetic subjects [124].

Therapeutic approaches that were restricted to administration of growth factors [125], endothelial progenitor cells for issue reconstruction [126], or stem cells [127] have shown limited results. Enhanced by increased applications in nanotechnology, miRNA-based therapeutic strategies have tremendous potential without many side effects [128]. *In vitro* and *in vivo* success has been reported for selective knockout of specific miRNAs by using gene manipulation methods or antagomiRs [129, 130]. Several miRNAs with enhanced actions during DM or its complications, identified in mouse models of DM have potential as therapeutic targets [131]. Those miRNAs that have been targeted effectively in other pathological conditions have potential applications in DM. For instance improved repair of dermal wounds has been shown in miR-155 knockout mice [132]. Although its expression is not enhanced in DM patients, it plays an important role in inflammation and could be targeted to reduce inflammation in diabetic wounds.

Replenishment of miRNA holds promise as a novel therapeutic strategy, when difficulties associated with tissue specificity and *in vivo* delivery methods are overcome [133]. Their high redundancy also makes it difficult to use miRNAs as therapeutic targets. It has been documented [134] that miR-146 is a good therapeutic target in DM, functioning as a molecular brake in stalling inflammation [135]. It appears to be significantly down-regulated in diabetic wounds in mouse models [136]. MiR-146 down-regulates the inflammatory markers IRAK-1 and TRAF-6; and cytokines (TNF-α, IL-6 and IL-1) [137]. Boosting miR-146 in mice also results in mimicry of autoimmune disorders akin to human autoimune lymphoproliferative syndrome [138]. In this context, treatment with mesenchymal stem cells proved to be more effective in upregulating miR-146a expression; and in promoting wound healing in a diabetic mouse model [136]. In view of these limitations, utilization of miRNAs as therapeutic targets for managing foot ulcers in DM remains a challenge. All diagnostic markers are potential therapeutic targets. For example, wound healing could be enhanced by promoting leukocyte migration to the site, attenuating bacterial infection and promoting wound closure. There is improved angiogenesis and activation of fibroblasts and keratinocytes via upregulation of miR-21 and mi-R-126. Downregulation of miR-203 and miR-210 which promote keratinocyte migration and proliferation would also enhance wound healing.

MiRNAs are involved in regulating and refining several pathophysiological processes in human diseases. They have a fascinating spectrum of such activities in RNA biology; applicable to wound healing in DM, activation of specific signalling pathways and modulation of gene expression pathways in response to stimuli. Some miRNA molecules provide valuable clinical information. They could potentially be tapped as early predictive diagnostic tools, for screening high risk subjects; thus aiding the decision-making process. The results of large-scale screening studies and those arising from *in vitro* cell systems, would require validation of markers in an *in vivo* environment. This would be a test of their functionality in a working environment, comprising tremendous diversity of interactions and overlap. It could detract from results obtained in a purer setting, *in vitro*. Each of these facets of information would constitute the larger picture. Critical knowledge of the pathways involved and functions that are as yet unknown, would contribute towards unravelling the mysteries of miRNAs. Tissue-specific actions of miRNAs and the effects of prevailing conditions on their expression, make it more complex. However, when they are validated *in vivo*, they could be effective therapeutic targets.

The single stranded non-coding miRNAs regulate gene expression at the post-transcriptional level. They bind to untranslated regions (UTR) of target mRNAs which leads to attenuated expression of target genes. It has been documented that miRNAs are universally involved in genetic pathways which underscores their importance in regulating pathophysiological processes. Regulatory small molecules hold promise as effective probes for exploration of the regulatory network mediated by miRNAs. Specific and universal small-molecule regulators of miRNAs associated with diseases, have been documented to have potential applications as therapeutic agents; based on screening systems developed fairly recently [139].

Improved outcome in surgical reconstructive procedures and regenerative medicine could be enhanced by inducible systems. They provide precise modulation of spatial and temporal control of differentiation, in tissue regenerative procedures. The effects of nanoformulated miRNA conjugates activated by photo exposure, on the induced osteogenic differentiation of human adipose-derived stromal stem cells (hASCs), have been studied *in vivo* [140]. A conjugated mimetic of miRNA-148 attached to silver nanoparticles (SNPs) via a photolabile linker, was used to modulate gene expression; for enhanced closure of an induced critical size parietal bone defect, in CD-1 nude homozygous mice. Varying degrees of healing were seen, when the conjugates added to hASCs were loaded onto Matrigel or polycaprolactone (PCL) scaffolds. Defect closure was statistically significant for both photoactivated and non-photoactivated conjugates loaded on PCL scaffolds at 4 and 12 weeks. Collagen fibre staining peaked at 12 weeks when it acquired the same density and consistency as the original calvarium. This model demonstrates the efficacy of the technology used, providing a platform for further applications; with other miRNAs that actively influence pathways governing wound healing and regeneration. An endogenous negative feedback mechanism for translation of mRNA to protein, is provided by noncoding miRNAs. Regulation of a range of mRNAs by single miRNAs, results in robust coordinated biological activity, impacting on multiple gene networks. Recent therapeutic applications for improved tissue repair/regeneration, using tools available for miRNA inhibition are addressed in a review [141].

The current gold standards for healing and regeneration of critical size bone defects (CSD), that do not heal spontaneously during the lifetime of an animal, are osteoinductive/osteoconductive autografts. They are often compromised by limited supply, donor site morbidity and infection. There is tremendous scope for bone tissue engineering in regenerating CSDs [142, 143]. Improved bone regeneration could be achieved with scaffolds for the delivery of therapeutic agents and proteins; including angiogenic and osteogenic factors, that enhance the expression of bone morphogenetic proteins (BMPs) [144] and vascular endothelial growth factor [145, 146, 147]. Over-expression or inhibition of miRNAs, offers potential advantages over the delivery of single proteins, in regulating the endogenous expression of multiple growth factors simultaneously [148]. Optimally coordinated angiogenesis and osteogenesis could be induced by modulating specific miRNAs [149]. Fracture healing and neovascularisation have been shown to occur in trochanteric fractures in response to down-regulation of miR-92a [150]. MiR-92a is considered to be an inhibitor of angiogenesis [151]. Inhibition of miRNA is a powerful tool, for enhanced mesenchymal stem cell function in tissue engineered constructs, in addition to coordinating angiogenesis [152].

It is relevant that the osteogenic potential of bone mesenchymal stem cells is significantly increased in response to inhibition of endogenous miR-31. When bone marrow stem cells (BMSCs) were lentivirally-transfected to express anti-miR-31, there was a 2.5-fold increase in the expression of AT-rich sequence-binding protein 2 which is involved in differentiation of osteoblasts and bone formation [153]. The increased expression of this protein was maintained at a constant level, upto 21 days after induction.The applications of miR-31 modulated activity in BMSCs, pertaining to critical size bone defects *in vivo* were subsequently tested. BMSCs transfected *in vitro* with vectors containing anti-miR-31, were seeded on polyglycerol sebacate scaffolds and implanted in rat calvarial critical size defects of 8mm. When examined at 8 weeks, there was significantly greater bone regeneration in critical size defects, when anti-miR-31 pre-treated cells were used in the scaffolds, over scaffolds alone. This indicates a role for anti-miRNAs as effective therapeutic agents, for improved tissue integration and regeneration, via engineered constructs for bone regeneration.

Increasing potential for tissue engineering, via manipulation of genes through miRNAs is documented. Clinical applications have been significantly limited by a dearth in adequate site-specific, bioactive delivery systems. A novel system that accommodates a range of therapeutic applications has been developed, comprising a non-viral platform for miRNA mimics and antagomiRNAs. Effective delivery of mature miRNA molecues has been achieved by combining nanohydroxyapatite particles with reporter nano miRNAs and collagen-nanaohydroxyapatite scaffolds [154]. By doing so, this work accomplished the first non-viral, non-lipid platform with minimal treatment-associated cytotoxicity; for effective delivery of mature miRNA molecules to human mesenchymal stem cells (hMSCs). They are a particularly difficult cell type to transfect. There was significant interfering activity from nano miRNA-mimics and nano antagomiRNAs of greater than 90%, following successful transfection of hMSCs, over a 7 day period. When applied to 3D scaffolds, significant RNA interference continued to be effective: 20% and 88% respectively for nano miRNA-mimics and nano antagomiRNAs. There were no cytotoxicity problems over a 7 day period. This miRNA-activated scaffold system has tremendous potential for tissue engineering applications, via effective delivery of miRNAs, in monolayer and on scaffolds.

Due to its versatile applications, there is increasing documentation of miRNA therapeutics in tissue engineering [155, 156]. Cell lineage commitment, differentiation, proliferation and apoptosis are some of the diverse physiological processes affected by miRNA-induced silencing [157]. In a therapeutic context, miRNAs have the capacity for targeting multiple proteins involved in coordinated cell function [158]. Conversely, the reverse is also true, in that each gene may be controlled by multiple miRNAs. This could prove more useful than previous tissue engineering strategies such as single gene therapy. It is therefore possible to modulate protein expression with focused specificity of miRNA therapy, by using mimics or antagomiRNAs respectively, for overexpression or inhibition of miRNAs. Due to poor intracellular cytosolic transmission and susceptibility to nucleases, focused delivery of miRNAs remains a challenge; for effective utilisation of the vast potential of miRNA interference therapy.

The beneficial effects of nHA particles and collagen-nHA scaffolds, as systems for delivery of miRNA therapeutics to hMSCs, underscore their potential for tissue engineering applications in the future. This is a novel model that confirms the ability of nano miRNA-mimics and nano antagomiRNAs, to modulate post-transcriptional gene regulation in hMSCs. It shows significant efficacy, in a minimally cytotoxic mode of low-dose, single applications for pronounced silencing activities. The delivery vectors used in this model show tremendous potential for supporting bioactivation of the complexes formed. Although initially modelled with bone regeneration in mind, the functional coordination of components used could be applied to other scaffold systems. They could incorporate a range of miRNAs that have a role in tissue engineering, for diverse applications.

Scarring is a physiological response to tissue injury in adults. Although scarring occurs in skin, it does not seem to affect the oral cavity. The fibrotic response in oral tissue is essentially fibroproliferative, largely deficient in myofibroblasts [159, 160]. Scarring is characterized by myofibroblasts containing abundant α-SMA (smooth muscle actin). Excessive scarring leads to progressive tissue damage which could contribute to organ failure and mortality. There is a large group of such diseases that cannot be treated [161]. Scarring occurs as a consequence of excessive remodelling of ECM, due to α-SMA expression in myofibroblasts located in connective tissues of adults. Gingival tissues do not succumb to scarring. Valuable insight into scarless repair, is gleaned from an understanding of different responses of skin and gingivae to fibrotic stimuli. In comparison with dermal fibroblasts, gingival fibrobasts are less responsive to TGF-β, due to their reduced expression and activity of focal adhesion kinase (FAK). It has been shown that gingival fibroblasts show reduced expression of miR-218 in comparison with dermal fibroblasts. FAK expression in gingival fibroblasts is elevated via an FAK/src-dependent mechanism when pre-miR-218 is conveyed to gingival fibroblasts. This results in induction of α-SMA by TGF-β [162]. There is increased expression of the deubiquitinase cezanne, a direct target of miR-218, in gingival fibroblasts, compared with dermal fibroblasts. FAK expression is enhanced by knockdown of cezanne in gingival fibroblasts, resulting in induction of α-SMA by TGF-β. These results indicate that myofibroblast differentiation induced by TGF-β, is regulated by miR-218 in fibroblasts via cezanne/FAK.

Connective tissue composition comprises ECM and fibroblasts [163]. It is hypothesized that fibroblasts from different tissues/organs have a distinct genetic pattern with specific cell differentiation in order to perform diverse functions. Scarless tissue repair in gingival fibroblasts in response to fibrogenic stimuli, compared with dermal fibroblasts, is governed by their differential responses. Accordingly, gingival fibroblasts are less responsive to the potent growth factor TGF-β [164] and to mechanical strain. Myofibroblast differentiation is significantly induced differentially by TGF-β, demonstrated by expression of α-SMA mRNA and protein in dermal fbroblasts; and not in gingival fibroblasts. TGF-β promotes collagen production and myofibroblast differentiation by cell adhesion via src/FAK [165]. Gingival fibroblasts are less adhesive to ECM, with reduced expression of FAK compared with dermal fibroblasts [166]. The differential adhesive capacity of dermal and gingival fibroblasts could account for their diverse responses [164, 166]. Further work is required to clarify the molecular basis for reduced expression of FAK; and reduced potential for induction of α-SMA expression by TGF-β, in gingival fibroblasts.

The small, non-coding miRNAs that modulate transcriptional and post-transcriptional genes represent an ancient regulatory component; well conserved during evolution. A range of miRNAs are dysregulated in fibrotic conditions [167]. The hypothesis that altered miRNA expression patterns, could dictate phenotypic differences between fibroblasts of gingival and dermal origin, has been addressed. It provides potential insight into the basis for scarless tissue repair, using gingival and dermal fibroblast models; demonstrating the relative inability of TGF-β to induce myofibroblast differentiation in gingival fibroblasts. This results in a hyperproliferative response in gingivae in response to stimuli, rather than scarring, due to the absence of highly contractile myofibroblasts.

In keeping with these findings, neither mechanical stress nor TGF-β can induce α-SMA in gingival fibroblasts, compared with dermal fibroblasts. This difference is due to diminished basal endothelin-1 (ET-1) production in gingival fibroblasts resulting from reduced FAK/src activity in these cells [164, 166]. These differences are bourne out in the raised adhesive signalling observed in dermal fibroblasts compared with those from gingivae. This appears to underpin diversity, in responses to TGF-β between these cell types. Reduced levels of miR-218 in gingival fibroblasts account for differential responses to TGF-β in gingival and dermal fibroblasts. Following post-differentiation of dental stem cells, interestingly miR-218 has been shown to be down-regulated [168] and attenuates proliferation of cancer cells [169]. The concept of the role of cezanne in the response of TGF-β or fibrosis has not been documented previously.

The fact that cezanne is also regulated by miR-486 is a significant finding of note [170]. These findings constitute important data suggesting mechanisms for scarless tissue repair, fundamentally based on epigenetic changes. They result in altered miR-218 expression, leading to reduced adhesive potential of gingival fibroblasts and altered TGF-β signalling.There are potential applications of these principles, for modulation of miR-218/cezanne or adhesive signalling, for the regulation of scarring in response to tissue injury.

Wound healing is a complex physiological response to tissue injury in an attempt to repair, in organ systems. It results in the formation of cytokines, growth factors and chemokines by damaged tissue. Identifying relevant biochemical pathways and cell types involved, is a crucial challenge. Several critical biological processes such as cell migration, proliferation, differentiation, activation and inhibition of signal pathways; and cell senescence are dictated by epigenetic mechanisms such as: DNA methylation, histone modification and editing of noncoding regulatory miRNAs [171]. Epigenetic regulators have potential for coordinated control of subsets of known repair genes. They mastermind a facet of wound healing. Epigenetic modifications could control pivotal gene expression and cell signal transduction for wound healing, in the short- and long-term. Therapeutic strategies based on epigenetics are directed at enhancing wound healing. They result in alteration of diverse cell types at sites of damage/injury; and induction of cell-signalling, leading to tissue repair. There is increasing documentation on the epigenetics of wound repair and processes involved.

Wound healing mechanisms involved are surprisingly generic involving diverse cell types, requiring the generation of fibrobasts, myofibroblasts and other cells, by a process of extensive alteration in gene expression. Thus cell phenotypes are regulated by a combination of molecular components of the epigenome. They comprise diverse post-translational modifications of chromatin components, DNA methylation and regulatory noncoding RNAs, such as miRNAs [167].

Epigenetic mechanisms regulate generation and apoptosis of myofibroblasts, in organs affected by disturbed healing. Some of these mechanisms are involved in fibrotic diseases. The therapeutic potential of epigenetic drugs and some miRNAs are being tested in this context. Epigenetic control mechanisms have scope for providing new developments in diagnostic, prognostic and wound healing applications. With the evolution of more specific epigenetic therapeutics, there would be greater control over optimal healing responses.

Differentiation of Human Dental Stem Cells (hDSCs) and a Role for miRNA in hDSCs

The ultimate goal of periodontal therapy is the regeneration of lost peridontium. The multilineage potential and plasticity of stem cells isolated from the periodontium have been demonstrated, due to advances in tissue engineering and regeneration. However, details of targeting tissue specificity and focus on cell lineage, by epigenetic mechanisms that control cell signalling, require further clarification. There is no available data on micro-RNA activity, driving dental stem cells (DSCs) derived from humans. Stem cells from human periodontal ligament, dental pulp and gingivae isolated from extracted third molars, were analysed for the expression of RUNX2, as a marker of mineralized tissue differentiation; following confirmation of OCT4A and NANOG transcription factor expression in these undifferentiated cells. Bone marrow stem cells were used as controls. Cells were cultured under conditions for induction of osteogenesis. The expression of miRNA was obtained at baseline and following osteogenic induction [168]. Effective osteogenic induction was demonstrated in all cells by RUNX2 expression. On analysing 765 miRNAs, there was a shift in miRNA expression in all 4 stem cell types including decreased has-mir-218 expression, across all differentiatied cells. RUNX2 is targeted by has-mir-218 and reduces its expression in undifferentiated human DSCs. Mineralised tissue type differentiation of DSCs is associated with reduced expression of hsa-mir- 218. This data indicates a microRNA- regulated pathway for human DSC differentiation, controlled by a specific network of miRNAs for osteogenic differentiation.

Adult stem cells of dental origin (DSC) derived from periodontal ligament (PDLSC), dental pulp (DPSC) and attached gingivae (GSC), provide a less invasive alternative source of stem cells when compared with bone marrow stem cells. They have the advantage of possessing similar properties [172, 173, 174, 175]. The status of differentiation of stem cells is influenced by a range of transcription factors. Tight regulation of the levels of OCT4 (octamer-binding transcription factor 4) is required, in order to maintain stem cell phenotype. Similarly another transcription factor NANOG, encoded by the NANOG gene is pivotal for maintaining the undifferentiated status of stem cells [176]. There is parallel activity of NANOG with cytokine stimulation of STAT3, to direct self-renewal of embryonic stem cells. Runt-related transcription factor 2

(RUNX2), has been found to be critical for osteoblastic differentiation and skeletal morphogenesis. There is increased RUNX2/CBFA1 (core binding factor) activity in bone marrow stromal cells during osteoblast differentiation.

MiRNAs are a class of post-transcriptional regulators that bind to specific complementary sequences of target mRNAs. They have the capacity to bind 60% of all genes. Each miRNA has multiple target genes, which it could attenuate [177]. There are several murine miRNAs that regulate osteogenesis. Osteoblast differentiation is negatively regulated by miRNA-26a and miRNA-125b [178]; and positively regulated by miRNA-29b and miRNA-210 [179]. Several miRNA regulatory pathways for mouse osteoblast differentiation have been identified. These include a RUNX2/miRNA-3960/miRNA-2861 regulatory feedback loop [180] and transcriptional control of an miRNA-23a-27a-24-2 cluster involving SATB2, by Runx2 [181]. It has also been shown, that specific miRNAs target RUNX2 in human BMSCs (bone marrow stem cells) [182] and cell differentiation programmes of murine osteoblasts [183]. A unique relationship between human miRNAs is expressed in undifferentiated DSCs. Progressive differentiation of these cells towards mineralized tissue, has been identified and compared with a well-characterised BMSC model. It is significant that in a defined set of human miRNAs involved in this progression, there was a correlation between expression of RUNX2; and reduced expression of miRNA-218 in human differentiated DSCs.

The STRO-1 surface marker antibody has had consistent applications in identifying stromal cell precursors in human bone marrow. Characteristic RUNX2 expression and calcium deposits [184] are associated with STRO-1 positive cells which show plasticity towards differentiation into osteoprogenitor cell types [185]. STRO-1 is a reliable tool for isolating stem cells of dental origin [172]. Certain cells from a heterogenous population of dental pulp (DP), gingival tissue (GT) and periodontal ligament (PDL), bind the antibody. Additional stem cell markers used to identify these cells: CD105, CD29, SSEA4 and OCT4 [186, 187, 188], tally with the STRO-1-positive results. They compare favourably with other studies [172, 189], being lowest in dental pulp. The number of stem cells available at perivascular sites, is directly associated with age of the donor, which is difficult to ascertain from pooled samples. The expression of OCT4 and NANOG denotes undifferentiated cells. There is tight regulation of OCT4 expression in mouse embryonic stem cells in order to maintain the phenotype. Increased OCT3/4 expression results in differentiation into primitive endoderm and mesoderm. Their attenuation induces loss of pluripotency, resulting in de-differentiation to trophoectoderm. Similarly, the transcription factor NANOG is pivotal in maintaining stem cells in an undifferentiated state. NANOG plays a role in driving self-renewal of embryonic stem cells by acting in coordination with cytokine stimulation of STAT3. STRO-1 labelled DSCs express these transcription factors, when compared with well-characterised human bone marrow stem cells. This provides further confirmation of their undifferentiated status.

Induction of DSCs in order to enable cell signalling cascades, progresses to cell lineage differentiation. Cell culture of PDLSC, DPSC, GSC and BMSC under conditions for inducing osteogenesis results in the formation of mineral deposits [172, 189, 190]. Peak expression of the transcription factor RUNX2 was used to correlate temporal events with the greatest degree of osteogenic activity. RUNX2 initiates a cascade of cell signalling leading to cell differentiation. It promotes the expression of ECM products associated with mineralized tissue. RUNX2 plays a pivotal role in osteoblast differentiation [191]. It belongs to the RUNX family of transcription factors and the nuclear protein that it encodes, has a RuntDNA-binding domain. Peak expression of RUNX2 at 2-4 weeks for BMSCs, DPSCs, GSCs and PDLSCs, tallied with the results of previous studies. A mesodermal embryological niche of BMSCs could account for greater potential for mineralization, associated with early UNX2 expression in these cells; compared with the ectodermal origin of PDLSC, GSC and DPSC.

The profile of BMSCs shows that when they are induced to differentiate in osteogenic culture, eight miRNAs are down-regulated in these stem cells. Amongst these miRNAs, recent documentation also confirms down-regulation of hsa-miR-148a and hsa-miR-31in BMSCs [180]. This is suggestive of an important role, in inhibition of osteogenic differentiation of mesenchymal stem cells. These findings are confirmatory of the crucial role of these miRNAs in the sequence of osteogenesis. MiRNA profiles in human stem cells of dental origin have not been reported previously. Decreased expression of hsa-miRNA-210, hsa-miRNA-222, hsamiRNA-218 and hsa-miRNA-99a in DPSC, GSC and PDLSC during osteogenesis, helps to define their role in cell differentiation. They appear to play a crucial role in dental stem cell differentiation. However there was no overlap in the overall miRNA profiles of each of these cell types, despite their embryological origins being the same. These differential expressions of miRNAs may be accounted for, by a specific niche for each cell type within diverse tissues of dental origin, resulting in differential expression of miRNAs. It is relevant that hsa-miR-210 and hsa-miR-222 were also down-regulated in BMSCs, in addition to being expressed in both dental cell types. It is apparent that these miRNAs could play a crucial role in osteogenesis across diverse cell/tissue types. Further work would clarify mechanisms involved.

There is novel documentation of differential expression of human DSCs (dermal stem cells) during osteogenic differentiation. It shows that RUNX2 expression is targeted by human miRNA-218. A group of osteo-miRNAs including miRNA-218, has been shown to control osteogenic maturation by targeting RUNX2 in mesenchymal cells [181]. In view of variable repression of RUNX2 by these miRNAs, it has been suggested that increased expression of miRNA at a late stage of osteoblast differentiation, allows maturation by decreasing RUNX2 expression. There are diverse mechanisms regulating osteoblast differentiation via miRNA and RUNX2 expression. This is shown by a novel RUNX2/miRNA-3960/miRNA2861 regulatory feedback loop, demonstrating that these miRNAs play a role in the differentiation of osteoblasts.

Chapter 10

Three Dimensional (3D) Printing of Tissue Regenerative Materials and Their Applications

3D printing of tissue components such as cells and matrices, has been used for fabrication of tissue analogues. The efficacy of 3D-printed biomimetic scaffolds conveying osteogenic factors, to promote healing in critical-sized mandibular defects has been studied in a novel animal model. A prospective animal study was carried out to study the efficacy of biomimetic PLGA scaffolds, to repair a critical-sized segmental mandibular defect in a rat model; alone and in combination with bone morphogenetic protein (BMP-2) and adipose-derived stem cells (ASCs) [192]. ASCs were isolated from the inguinal fat of rat pups. 3D printing was used to fabricate PLGA scaffolds which were impregnated with BMP-2 and or ASC. Blank PLGA scaffolds, PLGA scaffolds with ASCs, PLGA scaffolds impregnated with BMP or PLGA scaffolds with both BMP and ASCs, were implanted in adult rats, in 5mm critical-sized segmental mandibular defects that were created. Semi-quantitative bone formation and bone union scales were used to assess bone regeneration at 12 weeks, using microCT analysis. In rats implanted with blank scaffolds, there was no bridging of segmental bone defects, demonstrated by microCT analysis. Rats implanted with scaffolds containing BMP-2, ASCs and a combination of BMP and ASCs, showed healing of critical-sized segmental mandibular defects. Bone regeneration was most robust in the PLGA scaffolds treated with BMP-2.

There is intensive study of the development of a new generation of biomaterials for rapid osseointegration with host bone, with enhanced osteogenic capacity. A 3D printing technique is used to fabricate three dimensional mesoporous bioactive glass scaffolds, containing strontium (Sr-MBG). The physical characteristics of these scaffolds demonstrate interconnected macropores that are uniform with high porosity, and elevated compressive strength. The biological properties of Sr-MBG scaffolds were evaluated for characteristics of MC3T3-E1 osteoblast-like cells. Adhesion, proliferation, alkaline phosphatase activity, ability to form apatite and osteogenic gene expression of MC33-E1 were studied on Sr-MBG scaffolds, for comparison with MBG scaffolds, as controls [193]. The Sr-MBG scaffolds were also used to repair critical-sized rat calvarial defects. As evidenced by the results, Sr-MBG scaffolds are effective in forming apatite, with enhanced cell proliferation and differentiation of MC3T3-E1 osteoblast-like cells. It is significant that the *in vivo* results showed desirable osteogenic capacity of Sr-MBG scaffolds with enhanced induction of the formation of vasculature within 8 weeks, in these bone defects. 3D printed Sr-MBG scaffolds with favourable pore structure hold promise for further potential applications in bone regeneration, in view of their enhanced osteogenic capacity.

A guided bone regeneration (GBR) membrane has been fabricated by 3D printing consisting of polycaprolactone (PCL) / poly(lactic-co-glycolic acid) (PLGA) / β-TCP, designed for slow release of rh BMP-2 [194]. The GBR membrane was impregnated with intact rhBMP-2. In order to impregnate the membrane, rhBMP-2 was encapsulated in a collagen solution and infused into pores of the PCL/PLGA/βTCP membrane, fabricated using a 3D printing system with 4 dispensing heads. A release profile showed that there was sustained release of rhBMP-2 over a 28 day period. The efficacy of the GBR memebrane on bone regeneration was studied by implanting the PCL/PLGA/β-TCP membranes with or without rh BMP-2 in 8mm calvarial defects of rabbits. Space-making ability of the membrane was maintained successfully in both groups. Bone formation was analysed at 4 and 8 weeks using histological and histomorphometric evaluation. There was significantly greater bone formation, at post-implantation weeks 4 and 8 in response to rhBMP-2 loaded GBR membranes. Almost complete healing of the calvarial bone defect occurred at 8 weeks, in response to GBR membranes loaded with rhBMP-2.

A similar slow delivery system using human bone morphogenetic protein-2 (rhBMP-2) in PCL/poly(lactic-coglycolic acid) scaffolds produced by 3D printing, has been formulated successfully, for bone formation in critical sized diaphyseal defects of rabbits [195]. Temporal control of delivery of rhBMP-2 was achieved, by using collagen for long-term delivery over 28 days and gelatin for short-term delivery over one week. Solutions of collagen and gelatin encapsulating rhBMP-2, were dispensed at 5μg/ml in PCL/PLGA scaffolds that were hollow and cylindrical. The effective concentration was based on alkaline phosphatase and osteocalcin gene expression levels, in human mesenchymal stromal cells derived from human nasal inferior turbinate bones (hTMSCs); seeded on PCL/PLGA/collagen scaffolds (long-term) *in vitro*. It was observed that PCL/PLGA/gelatin scaffolds releasing a burst of rhBMP-2, at an equivalent dose in the short-term, did not induce osteogenic differentiation of hTMSCs *in vitro*. Using microcomputed tomography and histological analysis, the best quality of bone regeneration was found to occur, in response to the long-term delivery mode using PCL/PLGA/ collagen/rhBMP-2 scaffolds; at 4 and 8 weeks post-implantation. There was no inflammatory response. However, the short-term delivery model comprising PCL/PLGA/gelatin/rhBMP-2, generated a pronounced inflammatory response with a significant number of macrophages, during burst release of rhBMP-2 at week 4; indicating a superior response from the PCL/PLGA/collagen scaffold.

3D printing of calcium phosphate scaffolds at low temperature, has been proposed as a superior productive technique over traditional methods; for fabrication of synthetic bone graft substitutes [196]. Achieving optimal biocompatibility and osteoconductivity with good mechanical properties, requires detailed attention to design parameters; such as properties of binder solutions. A suitable concentration of phosphoric acid-based binder solution was used to maximize mechanical strength and cytocompatibility, supplemented with Tween 80 for enhanced printing. Dissolving collagen in the binder solution resulted in the formation of composites of collagen and calcium phosphate, thus further reinforcing the formulation. Using a physiological thermal treatment reduced viscosity; and the application of Tween 80, reduced surface tension. This results in reliable thermal inkjet printing of the collagen solutions. Supplementation of the binder solution with collagen of 1-2% by weight, significantly enhances cell viability and optimum flexural strength. 3D printed scaffolds were implanted for 9 weeks in critical sized murine femoral bone defects, in order to assess bone healing performance. It was confirmed that the implants were osteoconductive with osteogenesis around degrading scaffold material. This study demonstrates that optimising material parameters, by incorporating volumetric collagen for 3D inkjet printing of calcium phosphate scaffolds, enhances bone regeneration.

Tissue engineering as a strategy for bone regeneration and applications of bone grafts has been reviewed in the field of orthopaedic surgery. The pros and cons of bone grafting, analysing its characteristics, positive and limiting features are evaluated, incorporating discussion and elucidation of bone tissue engineering technologies [197]. Bone repair and regeneration are enhanced by a range of grafting materials comprising autografts, allografts and bone substitutes, used alone or in combination with each other. Autografts are considered to be the gold standard for these applications, as they include osteoconductive growth factors and allied agents. They provide osteogenic cells and a scaffold that is osteoconductive, essential for new growth formation. Autografts pose limited availability and an element of morbidity at the donor site, where bone is harvested. There is a risk of disease transmission, infection and rejection associated with allografts and xenografts. The newer and more progressive technological concepts associated with tissue engineering, overcome some of the limitations affecting the applications for bone grafting. There is potential for enhanced healing responses at bone defects and fractures. Combinations of scaffolds, regenerative agents, gene therapy and applications for 3D printing of constructs in tissue engineering, open avenues for exciting developments in the near future.

There is increasing popularity of techniques for 3D printing of tissue engineering constructs. They are fast becoming the cutting edge of procedures for tissue engineered regeneration of bone and soft tissue. There are increasing demands on clinicians regarding greater emphasis on patient centred care. Enhanced knowledge and scientific advancement of interactive technology, combining cells and biomaterials, has lead to greater specificity and focus; in streamlining cells for the delivery of bioactive nanoagents within definitive scaffold designs [198]. Effective formulation of scaffolds more readily, with multiple materials laden with appropriate cells, using the cutting edge technology of 3D printing, hold promise. The current status of 3D printing has been reviewed, with emphasis on producing nanomaterials; and their complex interactions with tissue engineered constructs for regenerative applications.

Bioactivity, bioresorbability and mechanical strength are required characteristics of the new generation of biomaterials for bone regenerative applications. Excellent bioactivity, biodegradability and drug delivery are some of the novel properties of mesoporous bioactive glass (MBG). They have been utilized to study bone regeneration [199]. However, their brittle characteristics and reduced strength pose challenges for the construction of 3D scaffolds for applications in bone regeneration. A relatively simple method for the preparation of a multifunctional MBG, broken down into progressive components has been described. It maximizes mechanical strength, mineralizing ability and a pore architecture that can be controlled for applications in bone regeneration; using polyvinyl alcohol (PVA) as a binder, in a modified 3D printing method. The novel method used, helps to overcome common problems governing inorganic scaffold materials. They are characterised by poor strength and brittleness with pore architecture that cannot be controlled, requiring high temperature sintering to be repeated. The mechanical strength of 3D printed MBG scaffolds is about 200-fold greater, than the traditionally used polyurethane foam templates. They demonstrate a pore architecture that can be controlled very well, with an excellent ability to mineralize apatite and incorporate features of sustained drug delivery. The 3D printed MBG scaffolds using PVA as a binder, prepared successfully, have significant advantages for applications in bone regeneration. They contain well-distributed mesopores and a hierarchical pore architecture with a high compressive strength. The PVA binder provides significant strength with reduced brittleness. It provides a new way of solving problems associated with pore architecture, strength, brittleness and the need for a second sintering cycle, amongst inorganic biodegradable scaffold materials. These pronounced advantages of 3D printed MBG scaffolds, with an excellent ability for apatite mineralization and good capacity as carriers for sustained drug delivery; render ideal properties for bone regenerative and tissue engineering applications.

Conclusion

It is a challenge to replicate biologically functional tissue. Principles applied to periodontal regeneration, constitute an excellent model for strategies that can be applied to regenerative medicine. A multidisciplinary approach is required, incorporating molecular biology, material science, nanotechnology and bioengineering; for effective translation to functional tissues. Proof of principle coverage of clinical applications indicates feasibility of these concepts, for effective delivery and more consistent outcome. Isolation of postnatal stem cells from diverse sources in the oral cavity and the development of smart biomaterials for cell and growth factor delivery; provide novel, alternative options for bioengineering and therapeutics. For the regeneration of lost tissue, the classical tissue engineering components comprising stem cells, ECM, scaffold materials, appropriate growth and differentiation factors have more streamlined applications; with improved focus on the applications of knowledge and technology. Interdisciplinary approaches are needed to drive tissue regeneration, involving clinicians, biologists, stem cell researchers and material scientists. Subject variables which affect disease susceptibility and presentation are likely to determine treatment outcome. This accounts for variation in clinical responses to strategies that show efficacy in *ex vivo* and *in vivo* studies. Biosafety requirements and generation of interest, for suitable investment in their development and availability; would dictate routine use of strategies addressed. It is possible that cell therapy will be implemented in clinical practice as a routine technique in the future, when existing limitations are overcome.

References

[1] Tatullo, M., Marrelli, M., Paduano, F., (2015). The regenerative medicine in oral and maxillofacial surgery: The most important innovations in the clinical application of mesenchymal stem cells. *Int. J. Med. Sci.* 12, 72-77.

[2] Fitzpatrick, L.E., McDevitt, T.C., (2015). Cell-derived matrices for tissue engineering and regenerative medicine applications 1. *Biomater. Sci.* 3, 12-24.

[3] De Jong, O.G., Van Balkom, B.W., Schiffelers, R.M., Bouten, C.V., Verhaar, M.C., (2014). Extracellular vesicles: potential roles in regenerative medicine. *Front Immunol.* 5, 608. doi: 10.3389/fimmu.2014.00608. eCollection 2014.

[4] Marino, A., Filippeschi, C., Mattoli, V., Mazzolai, B, Ciofani, G., (2014). Biomimicry at the nanoscale: current research and perspectives of two-photon polymerization. *Nanoscale* Dec 18. [Epub ahead of print].

[5] Xiao, Y., (2014). Bone tissue engineering for dentistry and orthopaedics. *Biomed Res. Int.* 241067. doi: 10.1155/2014/241067. Epub 2014 Nov 26.

[6] Shi, M., Zhai, D., Zhao, L., Wu, C., Chang, J., (2014). Nanosized mesoporous bioactive glass/poly(lactic-co-glycolic Acid) composite-coated $CaSiO_3$ scaffolds with multifunctional properties for bone tissue engineering. *BioMed Res. Int.* 2014, http: //dx.doi.org/ 10.1155/ 2014/323046.

[7] Lohberger, B., Kaltenegger, H., Stuendl, N., Payer, M., Beate Rinner, B, Leithner, A., (2014). Effect of cyclic mechanical stimulation on the expression of osteogenesis genes in human intraoral mesenchymal

stromal and progenitor cells. *BioMed Res. Int.* 2014, http://dx.doi.org/10.1155/2014/189516.

[8] Sanz, A.R., Carrión, F.S., Chaparro, A.P., (2015). Mesenchymal stem cells from the oral cavity and their potential value in tissue engineering. *Periodontol.2000* 67, 251-67.

[9] Cochran, D.L., Cobb, C.M., Bashutski, J.D., Chun, Y.H., Lin, Z., Mandelaris, G., McAllister, B.S., Murakami, S., Rios, H.F., (2015). Emerging regenerative approaches for periodontal reconstruction: A consensus report from the AAP workshop. *J. Periodontol.* 86 (2 Suppl.) S153-6.

[10] Chen, F.M., Sun, H.H., Lu, H., Yu, Q., (2012). Stem cell-delivery therapeutics for periodontal tissue regeneration. *Biomaterials* 33, 6320-44.

[11] Talal, A., McKay, I.J., Tanner, K.E., Hughes, F.J., (2013). Effects of hydroxyapatite and PDGF concentrations on osteoblast growth in a nanohydroxyapatite-polylactic acid composite for guided tissue regeneration. *J. Mater. Sci. Mater. Med.* 24, 2211-21.

[12] Bosshardt, D.D., Stadlinger, B., Terheyden, H., (2015). Cell-to-cell communication - periodontal regeneration. *Clin. Oral Implants Res.* 26, 229-39.

[13] Somoza, R.A., Acevedo, C.A., Albornoz, F., Luz-Crawford, P., Carrión, F., Young, M.E., Weinstein-Oppenheimer, C., (2015). TGFβ3 secretion by three-dimensional cultures of human dental apical papilla mesenchymal stem cells. *J. Tissue Eng. Regen. Med.* Feb 18. doi: 10.1002/term.2004. [Epub ahead of print].

[14] Pilipchuk, S.P., Plonka, A.B., Monje, A., Taut, A.D., Lanis, A., Kang, B., Giannobile, W.V., (2015). Tissue engineering for bone regeneration and osseointegration in the oral cavity. *Dent Mater.* Feb 17. pii: S0109-5641(15)00020-2. doi: 10.1016/j.dental.2015.01.006. [Epub ahead of print].

[15] Horst, O.V., Chavez, M.G., Jheon, A.H., Desai, T., Klein, O.D., (2012). Stem cell and biomaterials research in dental tissue engineering and regeneration. *Dent. Clin. North Am.* 56, 495-520.

[16] Murray, P.E., (2012). Constructs and scaffolds employed to regenerate dental tissue. *Dent. Clin. North Am.* 56, 577-88.

[17] El-Shinnawi, U., Soory, M., (2014). Periodontal regenerative materials and their applications: Mechanisms of action. *Rec. Pat. Regen. Med.* 4, 103-119.

[18] Reynolds, M.A., Kao, R.T., Camargo, P.M., Caton, J.G., Clem, D.S., Fiorellini, J.P., Geisinger, M.L., Mills, M.P., Nares, S., Nevins, M.L., (2015). Periodontal regeneration: Intrabony defects: A consensus report from the AAP regeneration workshop. *J. Periodontol.* 86 (2 Suppl), S105-7.

[19] Ebell, M.H., Siwek, J., Weiss, B.D., Woolf, S.H., Susman, J., Ewigman, B., Bowman, M., (2004). Strength of Recommendation Taxonomy (SORT): A patient-centred approach to grading evidence in the medical literature. *Am. Fam. Physician* 69, 548-56.

[20] Grandin, H.M., Gemperli, A.C., Dard, M., (2012). Enamel matrix derivative: a review of cellular effects *in vitro* and a model of molecular arrangement and functioning. *Tissue Eng. Part B Rev.*18, 181-202.

[21] Al-Qattan, T., Soory, M., (2012). Anabolic actions of the regenerative agent enamel matrix derivative (EMD) in oral periosteal fibroblasts and MG 63 osteoblasts; modulation by nicotine and glutathione in a redox environment. Special Issue on Biomaterials for Bone Substitutes. *J. Funct. Biomater.* 3, 143-162.

[22] Suchak, A., Soory, M., (2013). Anabolic potential of bone mineral in human periosteal fibroblasts using steroid markers of healing. *Steroids* 78, 462-67.

[23] Kao, R.T., Nares, S., Reynolds, M.A., (2015). Periodontal Regeneration-Intrabony Defects: A Systematic Review from the AAP Regeneration Workshop. *J. Periodontol.* 86 (2 Suppl), S77-104.

[24] Ivanovic, A., Nikou, G., Miron, R.J., Nikolidakis, D., Sculean, A., (2014). Which biomaterials may promote periodontal regeneration in intrabony periodontal defects? A systematic review of preclinical studies. *Quintessence Int.* 45, 385-95.

[25] Miron, R.J, Guillemette, V., Zhang,Y., Chandad, F., Sculean, A., (2014). Enamel matrix derivative in combination with bone grafts: A review of the literature. *Quintessence Int.* 45, 475-87.

[26] AboElsaad, N.S., Soory, M., Gadalla, L.M., Ragab, L.I., Dunne, S., Zalata, K.R., Louca, C., (2009). Effect of soft laser and bioactive glass on bone regeneration in the treatment of bone defects (An experimental study*), Lasers Med. Sci.* 24, 527-33.

[27] AboElsaad, N.S., Soory, M., Gadalla, L.M., Ragab, L.I., Dunne, S., Zalata, K.R., Louca, C., (2009). Effect of soft laser and bioactive glass on bone regeneration in the treatment of infrabony defects (A clinical study). *Lasers Med. Sci.* 24, 387-95.

[28] Panda, S., Doraiswamy, J., Malaiappan, S., Varghese, S.S., Del Fabbro, M., (2014). Additive effect of autologous platelet concentrates in treatment of intrabony defects: a systematic review and meta-analysis. *J. Investig. Clin. Dent.* Jul 22. doi: 10.1111/jicd.12117. [Epub ahead of print].

[29] Yan, X.Z., van den Beucken, J.J., Ca, X., Yu, N., Jansen, J.A., Yang, F., (2014). Periodontal tissue regeneration using enzymatically solidified chitosan hydrogels with or without cell Loading. *Tissue Eng. Part A*. Oct 25 [Epub ahead of print].

[30] Yan, X.Z., Nijhuis, A.W., van den Beucken, J.J., Both, S.K., Jansen, J.A., Leeuwenburgh, S.C., Yang, F., (2014). Enzymatic control of chitosan gelation for delivery of periodontal ligament cells. *Macromol. Biosci.* 14, 1004-14.

[31] Yan, X.Z., Both, S.K., Yang, P.S., Jansen, J.A., van den Beucken, J.J., Yang, F., (2014). Human periodontal ligament derived progenitor cells: effect of STRO-1 cell sorting and Wnt3a treatment on cell behavior. *Biomed Res. Int.* 2014:145423. doi: 10.1155/2014/145423. Epub 2014 Apr 28.

[32] Tatakis, D.N, Chambrone, L., Allen, E.P., Langer, B., McGuire, M.K., Richardson, C.R., Zabalegui, I., Zadeh, H.H., (2014). Periodontal soft tissue root coverage procedures: A consensus report. *J. Periodontol.* Oct 15, 1-6. [Epub ahead of print].

[33] Tonetti, M.S., Jepsen, S., (2014). Working Group 2 of the European Workshop on Periodontology. Clinical efficacy of periodontal plastic surgery procedures: consensus report of Group 2 of the 10th European Workshop on Periodontology. *J. Clin. Periodontol.* 41 Suppl. 15, S36-43.

[34] Aroca, S., Molnár, B., Windisch, P., Gera, I., Salvi, G.E., Nikolidakis, D., Sculean, A., (2013). Treatment of multiple adjacent Miller class I and II gingival recessions with a modified coronally advanced tunnel (MCAT) technique and a collagen matrix or palatal connective tissue graft: a randomized, controlled clinical trial. *J. Clin. Periodontol.* 40,713-20.

[35] Soory, M., (2008). Periodontal regenerative materials and their applications: Goodness of fit? *Recent Pat. Endocr. Metab. Immune Drug Discov*. 2, 35-44.

[36] Soory, M., (2011). In: *Wound Healing: Process, Phases and Promoting*. Healing in Periodontal bone defects: A Role for promoters? Nova

Science Publishers, Inc. Ed. Jane E Middleton. Chapter 1, p1-24. ISBN: 978-1-61209-847-0.

[37] Aguilera, V., Briceño, L., Contreras, H., Lamperti, L., Sepúlveda, E., Díaz-Perez, F., León, M., Veas, C., Maura, R., Toledo, J.R., Fernández, P., Covarrubias, A., Zuñiga, F.A., Radojkovic, C., Escudero, C., Aguayo, C., (2014). Endothelium trans- differentiated from Wharton's jelly mesenchymal cells promote tissue regeneration: Potential role of soluble pro-angiogenic factors. *PLoS One* 9, e111025. doi: 10.1371/journal.pone.0111025. eCollection 2014.

[38] Liu, S., Hou, K.D., Yuan, M., Peng, J., Zhang, L., Sui, X., Zhao, B., Xu, W., Wang, A., Lu, S., Guo, Q., (2014). Characteristics of mesenchymal stem cells derived from Wharton's jelly of human umbilical cord and for fabrication of non-scaffold tissue-engineered cartilage. *J. Biosci. Bioeng.* 117, 229-35.

[39] Compton, J.T., Lee, F.Y., (2014). A review of osteocyte function and the emerging importance of sclerostin. *J. Bone Joint Surg. Am.* 96, 1659-68.

[40] Sapir-Koren, R., Livshits, G., (2014). Osteocyte control of bone remodeling: is sclerostin a key molecular coordinator of the balanced bone resorption-formation cycles? *Osteoporos. Int.* 25, 2685-700.

[41] Bellido, T., (2014). Osteocyte-driven bone remodelling. *Calcif. Tissue Int.* 94, 25-34.

[42] Kubota, S., Takigawa, M., (2015). Cellular and molecular actions of CCN2/CTGF and its role under physiological and pathological conditions. *Clin Sci (Lond).* 128, 181-96.

[43] Xu, J., Huang, Z., Lin, L., Fu, M., Song, Y., Shen, Y., Ren, D., Gao, Y., Su, Y., Zou, Y., Chen, Y., Zhang, D., Hu, W., Qian, J., Ge, J., (2015). miRNA-130b is required for the ERK/FOXM1 pathway activation-mediated protective effects of isosorbide dinitrate against mesenchymal stem cell senescence induced by high glucose. *Int. J. Mol. Med.* 35, 59-71.

[44] Mahajan, A., (2012). Periosteum: A highly underrated tool in Dentistry. *Int. J. Dent.* 717816.

[45] Evans, S.F., Chang, H., Knothe Tate, M.L., (2013). Elucidating multiscale periosteal mechanobiology: a key to unlocking the smart properties and regenerative capacity of the periosteum? *Tissue Eng.Part B Rev.* 19, 147-59.

[46] Ferretti C, Mattioli-Belmonte M., (2014). Periosteum derived stem cells for regenerative medicine proposals: Boosting current knowledge. *World J. Stem Cells* 6, 266-77.

[47] Olivos-Meza, A., Fitzsimmons, J.S., Casper, M.E., Chen, Q., An, K-N., Ruesink, T.J., O'Driscoll, S.W., Reinholz, G.G., (2010). Pretreatment of periosteum with TGF-β1 *in situ* enhances the quality of osteochondral tissue regenerated from transplanted periosteal grafts in adult rabbits. *Osteoarthritis Cartilage* 18, 1183–1191.

[48] Uematsu, K., Kawase, T., Nagata, M., Suzuki, K., Okuda, K., Yoshie, H., Burns, D.M., Takagi, R., (2013). Tissue culture of human alveolar periosteal sheets using a stem-cell culture medium (MesenPRO-RS™): In vitro expansion of CD146-positive cells and concomitant upregulation of osteogenic potential *in vivo*. *Stem Cell Res.* 10, 1-19.

[49] Syed-Picard, F.N., Shah, G.A., Costello, B.J., Sfeir, C., (2014). Regeneration of periosteum by human bone marrow stromal cell sheets. *J. Oral Maxillofac. Surg.* 72, 1078-83.

[50] Baharvand, M., Mortazavi, A., Mortazavi, H., Yaseri, M., (2014). Re-evaluation of the first phenytoin paste healing effects on oral biopsy ulcers. *Ann. Med. Health Sci. Res.* 4, 858-62.

[51] Suchak, A., Soory, M., (2014). Biomarkers of regenerative responses to phenytoin in periosteal fibroblasts and modulation by histamine; relevance to inflammatory repair. *Rec. Pat. Biomarkers* 4, 163-172.

[52] Chang, H., Knothe Tate, M.L., (2012). Concise review: the periosteum: tapping into a reservoir of clinically useful progenitor cells. *Stem Cells Transl. Med.* 1, 480-91.

[53] Colnot, C., Zhang, X., Knothe Tate, M.L., (2012). Current insights on the regenerative potential of the periosteum: molecular, cellular, and endogenous engineering approaches. *J. Orthop. Res.* 30, 1869-78.

[54] Lin, Z., Fateh, A., Salem, D.M., Intini, G., (2014). Periosteum: biology and applications in craniofacial bone regeneration. *J. Dent. Res.* 93,109-16.

[55] Furth, M.E., Atala, A., Van Dyke, M.E., (2015). Smart biomaterials design for tissue engineering and regenerative medicine. *Biomed. Mater. Eng.* 25, 79-85.

[56] Toh, W.S, Loh, X.J., (2014). Advances in hydrogel delivery systems for tissue regeneration. *Mater Sci Eng. C Mater. Biol. Appl.* 45C, 690-97.

[57] Prestwich, G.D., Healy, K.E., (2015). Why regenerative medicine needs an extracellular matrix. *Expert Opin. Biol. Ther.* 15, 3-7.

[58] Lin, C., Ki, C.S., Shih, H., (2015). Thiol-norbornene photo-click hydrogels for tissue engineering applications. *J. Appl. Polym. Sci.* 132, pii: 41563.

[59] Ma, J., Yang, F., Both, S.K., Kersten-Niessen, M., Bongio, M., Pan, J., Cui, F.Z., Kasper, F.K., Mikos, A.G., Jansen, J.A., van den Beucken, J.J., (2014). Comparison of cell-loading methods in hydrogel systems. *J. Biomed. Mater. Res. A.* 102, 935-46.

[60] Yan, X.Z., van den Beucken, J.J., Both, S.K., Yang, P.S., Jansen, J.A., Yang, F., (2014). Biomaterial strategies for stem cell maintenance during in vitro expansion. *Tissue Eng. Part B Rev.* 20, 340-54.

[61] McMurray, R.J., Dalby, M.J., Tsimbouri, P.M., (2014). Using biomaterials to study stem cell mechanotransduction, growth and differentiation. *J. Tissue Eng. Regen. Med.* Nov 5. doi: 10.1002/term.1957. [Epub ahead of print].

[62] Gillette, B.M., Jensen, J.A., Wang, M., Tchao, J., Sia, S.K., (2010). Dynamic hydrogels: switching of 3D microenvironments using two-component naturally derived extracellular matrices. *Adv. Mater.* 22, 686-691.

[63] Yoshikawa, H.Y., Rossetti, F.F., Kaufmann, S., Kaindl, T., Madsen, J., Engel, U., Lewis, A.L., Armes, S.P., Tanaka, M., (2011). Quantitative evaluation of mechanosensing of cells on dynamically tunable hydrogels. *J. Am. Chem. Soc.* 133, 1367–1374.

[64] Le, D.M., Kulangara, K., Adler, A.F., Leong, K.W., Ashby, V.S., (2011). Dynamic topographical control of mesenchymal stem cells by culture on responsive poly(ε-caprolactone) surfaces. *Adv. Mater.* 23, 3278–3283.

[65] Ebara, M., Uto, K., Idota, N., Hoffman, J.M., Aoyagi, T., (2012). Shape-memory surface with dynamically tunable nano-geometry activated by body heat. *Adv. Mater.* 24, 273–278.

[66] Yeo, W.S., Hodneland,C.D., Mrksich, M., (2001). Electroactive monolayer substrates that selectively release adherent cells. *Chembiochem.* 2, 590–593.

[67] Yeo, W.S., Mrksich, M., (2006). Electroactive self-assembled monolayers that permit orthogonal control over the adhesion of cells to patterned substrates. *Langmuir* 22, 10816-10820.

[68] Wirkner, M., Weis, S., San Miguel, V., Álvarez, M., Gropeanu, R.A., Salierno, M., Sartoris, A., Unger, R.E., Kirkpatrick, C.J., del Campo, A., (2011). Photoactivatable caged cyclic RGD peptide for triggering integrin binding and cell adhesion to surfaces. *Chembiochem.* 12, 2623-2629.

[69] Todd, S.J., Farrah, D., Gough, J.E., Ulijn, R.V., (2007). Enzyme-triggered cell attachment to hydrogel surfaces. *Soft Matter* 3, 547–550.

[70] Todd, S.J., Scurr, D.J., Gough, J.E., Alexander, M.R., Ulijn, R.V., (2009). Enzyme activated RGD ligands on functionalized PEG monolayers: surface analysis and cellular response. *Langmuir* 25, 7533–7539.

[71] Brown, P.T., Handorf, A.M., Jeon, W.B., Li, W.J., (2013). Stem cell-based tissue engineering approaches for musculoskeletal regeneration. *Curr. Pharm. Des.*19, 3429-45.

[72] Kilian, K.A., Bugarija, B., Lahn, B.T., Mrksich, M., (2010). Geometric cues for directing the differentiation of mesenchymal stem cells. *Proc. Natl. Acad. Sci. USA*. 107, 4872–7.

[73] Huang, C.H., Chen, M.H., Young, T.H., Jeng, J.H., Chen, Y.J., (2009). Interactive effects of mechanical stretching and extracellular matrix proteins on initiating osteogenic differentiation of human mesenchymal stem cells. *J. Cell Biochem.* 108, 1263-73.

[74] Liu, L., Yuan, W., Wang, J., (2010). Mechanisms for osteogenic differentiation of human mesenchymal stem cells induced by fluid shear stress. *Biomech. Model Mechanobiol.* 9, 659–70.

[75] Liu, L., Yu, B., Chen, J., Tang, Z., Zong, C., Shen, D., Zheng, Q., Tong, X., Gao, C., Wang, J., (2012). Different effects of intermittent and continuous fluid shear stresses on osteogenic differentiation of human mesenchymal stem cells. *Biomech. Model Mechanobiol.* 11, 391–401.

[76] Yourek, G., McCormick, S.M., Mao, J.J., Reilly, G.C., (2010). Shear stress induces osteogenic differentiation of human mesenchymal stem cells. *Regen. Med.* 5, 713–24.

[77] Nöth, U., Rackwitz, L., Steinert, A.F., Tuan, R.S., (2010). Cell delivery therapeutics for musculoskeletal regeneration. *Adv. Drug Deliv. Rev.* 62, 765-83.

[78] Fang, Y., Chen, X., Wt, G., (2014). Gene delivery in tissue engineering and regenerative medicine. *J. Biomed. Mater. Res. B Appl. Biomater.* Dec 30. doi: 10.1002/jbm.b.33354. [Epub ahead of print].

[79] Kwiatkowski, W., Gray, P.C., Choe, S., (2014). Engineering TGF-β superfamily ligands for clinical applications. *Trends Pharmacol. Sci.* 35, 648-657.

[80] Han, P., Ivanovski, S., Crawford, R., Xiao, Y., (2015). Activation of the canonical Wnt signalling pathway induces cementum regeneration. *J. Bone Miner. Res.*Jan 1. doi: 10.1002/jbmr.2445. [Epub ahead of print].

[81] Nguyen, A.H., McKinney, J., Miller, T., Bongiorno, T., McDevitt, T.C., (2014). Gelatin methacrylate microspheres for controlled growth factor

release. *Acta Biomater.* Nov 20. pii: S1742-7061(14)00522-4. doi: 10.1016/j.actbio.2014.11.028. [Epub ahead of print].

[82] Suliman, S., Xing, Z., Wu, X., Xue, Y., Pedersen, T.O., Sun, Y., Døskeland, A.P., Nickel, J., Waag, T., Lygre, H., Finne-Wistrand, A., Steinmüller-Nethl, D., Krueger, A., Mustafa, K., (2015). Release and bioactivity of bone morphogenetic protein-2 are affected by scaffold binding techniques *in vitro* and *in vivo*. *J. Control. Release* 197, 148-57.

[83] Samorezov, J.E., Alsberg, E., (2014). Spatial regulation of controlled bioactive factor delivery for bone tissue engineering. *Adv. Drug Deliv. Rev.* Nov 29. pii: S0169-409X(14)00284-1. doi: 10.1016/j.addr. 2014.11.018. [Epub ahead of print].

[84] Hoogenkamp, H.R., Bakker, G.J., Wolf, L., Suurs, P., Dunnewind, B., Barbut, S., Friedl, P., van Kuppevelt, T.H., Daamen, W.F., (2015). Directing collagen fibers using counter-rotating cone extrusion. *Acta Biomater.* 12, 113-21.

[85] Marx, C., Silveira, M.D., Beyer Nardi N., (2015). Adipose-derived stem cells in veterinary medicine: characterization and therapeutic applications. *Stem Cells Dev.* Jan 4. [Epub ahead of print].

[86] Stoltz, J.F., Bensoussan, D., Zhang, L., Decot,V., De Isla, N., Li, Y.P., Huselstein, C., Benkirane-Jessel, N., Li, N., Reppel, L., He, Y., Li, Y.Y., (2015). Stem cells and applications: A survey. *Biomed. Mater. Eng.* 25, 3-26.

[87] Hewitt, K.J., Shamis, Y., Gerami-Naini, B., Garlick, J.A., (2014). Strategies for oral mucosal repair by engineering 3D tissues with pluripotent stem cells. *Adv. Wound Care* (New Rochelle) 3, 742-750.

[88] Yan, L.P., Silva-Correia, J., Oliveira, M.B., Vilela, C., Pereira, H., Sousa, R.A., Mano, J.F., Oliveira, A.L., Oliveira, J.M., Reis, R.L., (2015). Bilayered silk/silk-nanoCaP scaffolds for osteochondral tissue engineering: *In vitro* and *in vivo* assessment of biological performance. *Acta Biomater.* Jan 15;12:227-41. doi: 10.1016/j.actbio.2014.10.021. Epub 2014 Oct 23.

[89] Katti, D.R., Sharma, A., Ambre, A.H., Katti, K.S., (2015). Molecular interactions in biomineralized hydroxyapatite amino acid modified nanoclay: In silico design of bone biomaterials. *Mater. Sci. Eng. C Mater. Biol. Appl.* 46, 207-17.

[90] Ambre, A.H., Katti, D.R., Katti, K.S., (2014). Biomineralized hydroxyapatite nanoclay composite scaffolds with polycaprolactone for stem cell-based bone tissue engineering. J. *Biomed. Mater. Res. A.* Oct 21. doi: 10.1002/jbm.a.35342. [Epub ahead of print].

[91] Fan, J., Park, H., Lee, M.K., Bezouglaia, O., Fartash, A., Kim, J., Aghaloo, T., Lee, M., (2014). Adipose-derived stem cells and BMP-2 delivery in chitosan-based 3D constructs to enhance bone regeneration in a rat mandibular defect model. *Tissue Eng Part A*. 20, 2169-79.

[92] Gharibi, B., Ghuman, M.S., Hughes, F.J., (2012). Akt- and Erk-mediated regulation of proliferation and differentiation during PDGFRβ-induced MSC self-renewal. *J. Cell Mol. Med.* 16, 2789-801.

[93] Murayama, H., Masaki, H., Sato, H., Hayama, T., Yamaguchi, T., Nakauchi, H., (2014). Successful reprogramming of epiblast stem cells by blocking nuclear localization of β-catenin. *Stem Cell Reports* Dec 30. pii: S2213-6711(14)00360-9. doi: 10.1016/j.stemcr.2014.12.003. [Epub ahead of print].

[94] Langer, R., Tirrell, D.A., (2004). Designing materials for biology and medicine. *Nature* 428, 487-92.

[95] Weigel, T., Schinkel, G., Lendlein, A., (2006). Design and preparation of polymeric scaffolds for tissue engineering. *Expert Rev. Med. Devices* 3, 835–51.

[96] Tsang, V.L., Bhatia, S.N., (2007). Fabrication of three-dimensional tissues. *Adv. Biochem. Eng. Biotechnol.* 103, 189–205.

[97] Boccaccini, A.R., Blaker, J.J., (2005). Bioactive composite materials for tissue engineering scaffolds. *Expert Rev. Med. Devices.* 2, 303–17.

[98] Gharibi, B., Cama, G., Capurro, M., Thompson, I., Deb, S., Di-Silvio, L., Hughes, F.J., (2013). Gene expression responses to mechanical stimulation of mesenchymal stem cells seeded on calcium phosphate cement. *Tissue Eng. Part A.* 19, 2426-2438.

[99] Eap, S., Morand, D., Clauss, F., Huck, O., Stoltz, J.F., Lutz, J.C., Gottenberg, J.E., Benkirane-Jessel, N., Keller, L., Fioretti, F., (2015). Nanostructured thick 3D nanofibrous scaffold can induce bone. *Biomed. Mater. Eng.* 25 (1 Suppl), 79-85.

[100] Beachley, V., Kasyanov, V., Nagy-Mehesz, A., Norris, R., Ozolanta, I., Kalejs, M., Stradins, P., Baptista, L., da Silva, K., Grainjero, J., Wen, X., Mironov, V., (2014). The fusion of tissue spheroids attached to pre-stretched electrospun polyurethane scaffolds. *J. Tissue Eng.* Nov 6; 5:2041731414556561. doi: 10.1177/2041731414556561. eCollection 2014.

[101] Stoppel, W.L., Ghezzi, C.E., McNamar, S.L., Iii, L.D., Kaplan, D.L., (2014). Clinical applications of naturally derived diopolymer-based scaffolds for regenerative medicine. *Ann. Biomed. Eng.* Dec 24. [Epub ahead of print].

[102] Rnjak-Kovacina, J., Wray, L.S., Golinski, J.M., Kaplan, D.L., (2014). Arrayed hollow channels in silk-based scaffolds provide functional outcomes for engineering critically-sized tissue constructs. *Adv. Funct. Mater.* 24, 2188-2196.

[103] Kang, Y., Mochizuki, N., Khademhosseini, A., Fukuda, J., Yang, Y., (2015). Engineering a vascularized collagen-β-tricalcium phosphate graft using an electrochemical approach. *Acta Biomater.* 11, 449–458.

[104] Cuchiara, M.P., Gould, D.J., McHale, M.K., Dickinson, M.E., West, J.L., (2012). Integration of self assembled microvascular networks with microfabricated PEG-based hydrogels. *Adv. Funct.Mater.* 22, 4511–8.

[105] Chen, Y.C., Lin, R.Z., Qi, H., Yang, Y., Bae, H., Melero-Martin, J.M., Khademhosseini, A., (2012). Functional human vascular network generated in photocrosslinkable gelatin methacrylate hydrogels. *Adv. Funct.Mater.* 22, 2027–39.

[106] Beier, J.P., Horch, R.E., Hess, A., Arkudas, A., Heinrich. J, Loew J., Gulle, H., Polykandriotis, E., Bleiziffer, O., Kneser, U., (2010). Axial vascularization of a large volume calcium phosphate ceramic bone substitute in the sheep AV loop model. *J. Tissue Eng. Regen. Med.* 4, 216–23.

[107] Novosel, E.C., Kleinhans, C., Kluger, P.J., (2011). Vascularization is the key challenge in tissue engineering. *Adv. Drug Deliv. Rev.* 63, 300-11.

[108] Zhou, J., Lin, H., Fang, T., Li, X., Dai, W., Uemura, T., Dong, J., (2010). The repair of large segmental bone defects in the rabbit with vascularized tissue engineered bone. *Biomaterials* 31, 1171-9.

[109] Wang, L., Fan, H., Zhang, Z-Y., Lou, A-J., Pei, G-X., Jiang, S., Mu, T.W., Qin, J.J., Chen, S.Y., Jin, D., (2010). Osteogenesis and angiogenesis of tissue-engineered bone constructed by prevascularized btricalcium phosphate scaffold and mesenchymal stem cells. *Biomaterials* 31, 9452-61.

[110] Chiu, L.L., Montgomery, M., Liang, Y., Liu, H., Radisic, M., (2012). Perfusable branching microvessel bed for vascularization of engineered tissues. *Proc. Natl. Acad. Sci. USA*.109, E3414–23.

[111] Miller, J.S., Stevens, K.R,, Yang, M.T., Baker, B.M., Nguyen, D-HT., Cohen, DM., Toro, E., Chen, A.A., Galie, P.A., Yu, X., Chaturvedi, R., Bhatia, S.N., Chen, C.S., (2012). Rapid casting of patterned vascular networks for perfusable engineered three dimensional tissues. *Nat. Mater.* 11, 768–74.

[112] Visconti, R.P., Kasyanov, V., Gentile, C., Zhang, J., Markwald, R.R., Mironov, V., (2010). Towards organ printing: engineering an intra-organ branched vascular tree. *Expert Opin. Biol. Ther.* 10, 409–20.

[113] Zorlutuna, P., Annabi, N., Camci-Unal, G., Nikkhah, M., Cha, J.M., Nichol, J.W., Manbachi, A., Bae, H., Chen, S., Khademhosseini, A., (2012). Microfabricated biomaterials for engineering 3D tissues. *Adv. Mater.* 24, 1782–804.

[114] Nikkhah, M., Eshak, N., Zorlutuna, P., Annabi, N., Castello, M., Kim K., Dolatshahi-Pirouz, A., Edalat, F., Bae, H., Yang, Y., Khademhosseini, A., (2012). Directed endothelial cell morphogenesis in micropatterned gelatin methacrylate hydrogels. *Biomaterials* 33, 9009–18.

[115] Zheng, Y., Chen, J., Craven, M., Choi, N.W., Totorica, S., Diaz-Santana, A., Kermani, P., Hempstead, B., Fischbach-Teschl, C., López, J.A., Stroock, A.D., (2012). *In vitro* microvessels for the study of angiogenesis and thrombosis. *Proc. Natl. Acad. Sci. USA.* 109, 9342-7.

[116] Sadr, N., Zhu, M., Osaki, T., Kakegawa, T., Yang, Y., Moretti, M., Fukuda, J., Khademhosseini, A., (2011). SAM-based cell transfer to photopatterned hydrogels for microengineering vascular-like structures. *Biomaterials* 32, 7479–90.

[117] Mochizuki, N., Kakegawa, T., Osaki, T., Sadr, N., Kachouie, N.N., Suzuki, H., Fukuda, J., (2013). Tissue engineering based on electrochemical desorption of an RGD-containing oligopeptide. *J. Tissue Eng. Regen. Med.*7, 236–43.

[118] Eweida, A.M., Nabawi, A.S., Abouarab, M., Kayed, M., Elhammady, H., Etaby, A., Khalil, M.R., Shawky, M.S., Kneser, U., Horch, R.E., Nagy, N., Marei, M.K., (2014). Enhancing mandibular bone regeneration and perfusion via axial vascularization of scaffolds. *Clin. Oral Investig.*18, 1671-8.

[119] Moura, J., Børsheim, E., Carvalho, E., (2014). The role of microRNAs in diabetic complications-special emphasis on wound healing. *Genes (Basel).* 5, 926-56.

[120] Pottier, N., Maurin, T., Chevalier, B., Puissegur, M.P.; Lebrigand, K., Robbe-Sermesant, K., Bertero, T., Lino Cardenas, C.L., Courcot, E., Rios, G., Fourre, S., Lo-Guidice, J.M., Marcet, B., Cardinaud, B., Barbry, P., Mari, B., (2009). Identification of keratinocyte growth factor as a target of microRNA-155 in lung fibroblasts: Implication in epithelial-mesenchymal interactions. *PLoS ONE*, 4, e6718.

[121] Corral-Fernandez, N.E., Salgado-Bustamante, M., Martinez-Leija, M.E., Cortez-Espinosa, N., Garcia-Hernandez, M.H., Reynaga-Hernandez, E., Quezada-Calvillo, R., Portales-Perez, D.P., (2013). Dysregulated MIR-155 expression in peripheral blood mononuclear cells from patients with type 2 diabetes. *Exp. Clin. Endocrinol. Diabetes* 121, 347–353.

[122] Kishore, R., Verma, S.K., Mackie, A.R., Vaughan, E.E., Abramova, T.V., Aiko, I., Krishnamurthy, P., (2013). Bone marrow progenitor cell therapy-mediated paracrine regulation of cardiac miRNA-155 modulates fibrotic response in diabetic hearts. *PLoS One* 8, e60161.

[123] Madhyastha, R., Madhyastha, H.; Nakajima, Y., Omura, S., Maruyama, M., (2012). MicroRNA signature in diabetic wound healing: Promotive role of MIR-21 in fibroblast migration. *Int. Wound J.* 9, 355–361.

[124] Meng, S., Cao, J.T., Zhang, B., Zhou, Q., Shen, C.X., Wang, C.Q., (2012). Downregulation of microRNA-126 in endothelial progenitor cells from diabetes patients, impairs their functional properties, via target gene spred-1. *J. Mol. Cell Cardiol.* 53, 64–72.

[125] Game, F.L., Hinchliffe, R.J., Apelqvist, J., Armstrong, D.G., Bakker, K., Hartemann, A., Londahl, M., Price, P.E., Jeffcoate, W.J., (2012). A systematic review of interventions to enhance the healing of chronic ulcers of the foot in diabetes. *Diabetes Metab. Res. Rev.* 28, S119–S141.

[126] Sieveking, D.P., Ng, M.K., (2009). Cell therapies for therapeutic angiogenesis: Back to the bench. *Vasc. Med.* 14, 153–166.

[127] Kirana, S., Stratmann, B., Prante, C., Prohaska, W.; Koerperich, H., Lammers, D., Gastens, M.H., Quast, T., Negrean, M., Stirban, O.A., Nandrean S.G., Gotting, C., Minartz, P., Kleesiek, K., Tschoepe, D., (2012). Autologous stem cell therapy in the treatment of limb ischaemia induced chronic tissue ulcers of diabetic foot patients. *Int. J. Clin. Pract.* doi:10.1111/j.1742-1241.2011.02886.x.

[128] Shu, Y., Pi, F., Sharma, A., Rajabi, M., Haque, F., Shu, D., Leggas, M., Evers, B.M.; Guo, P., (2014). Stable RNA nanoparticles as potential new generation drugs for cancer therapy. *Adv. Drug Deliv. Rev.* 66, 74–89.

[129] Park, C.Y., Choi, Y.S., McManus, M.T., (2010). Analysis of microRNA knockouts in mice. *Hum. Mol. Genet.* 19, R169–R175.

[130] Ruberti, F., Barbato, C., Cogoni, C., (2012). Targeting microRNAs in neurons: Tools and perspectives. *Exp. Neurol.* 235, 419–426.

[131] Mori, M., Nakagami, H., Rodriguez-Araujo, G., Nimura, K., Kaneda, Y., (2012). Essential role for mir-196a in brown adipogenesis of white fat progenitor cells. *PLoS Biol.* 10, e1001314.

[132] Van Solingen, C., Araldi, E., Chamorro-Jorganes, A., Fernandez-Hernando, C., Suarez, Y., (2014). Improved repair of dermal wounds in mice lacking microRNA-155. *J. Cell Mol. Med.* doi:10.1111/jcmm.12255.

[133] Sakai, A., Saitow, F., Miyake, N., Miyake, K., Shimada, T., Suzuki, H., (2013). Mir-7a alleviates the maintenance of neuropathic pain through regulation of neuronal excitability. *Brain* 136, 2738–2750.

[134] Kovacs, B., Lumayag, S., Cowan, C., Xu, S., (2011). MicroRNAs in early diabetic retinopathy in streptozotocin-induced diabetic rats. *Invest. Ophthalmol. Vis. Sci.* 52, 4402–4409.

[135] Balasubramanyam, M., Aravind, S., Gokulakrishnan, K., Prabu, P., Sathishkumar, C., Ranjani, H., Mohan, V., (2011). Impaired MIR-146a expression links subclinical inflammation and insulin resistance in type 2 diabetes. *Mol. Cell Biochem.* 351, 197–205.

[136] Xu, J., Wu, W., Zhang, L., Dorset-Martin, W., Morris, M.W., Mitchell, M.E.; Liechty, K.W., (2012). The role of microRNA-146a in the pathogenesis of the diabetic wound-healing impairment: Correction with mesenchymal stem cell treatment. *Diabetes* 61, 2906–2912.

[137] Alipour, M.R., Khamaneh, A.M., Yousefzadeh, N., Mohammad-nejad, D., Soufi, F.G., (2013). Upregulation of microRNA-146a was not accompanied by downregulation of pro-inflammatory markers in diabetic kidney. *Mol. Biol. Rep.* 40, 6477–6483.

[138] Guo, Q., Zhang, J., Li, J., Zou, L., Zhang, J., Xie, Z., Fu, X., Jiang, S., Chen, G., Jia, Q., Li,F., Wan, Y., Wu, Y., (2013). Forced mir-146a expression causes autoimmune lymphoproliferative syndrome in mice via downregulation of fas in germinal center B cells. *Blood* 121, 4875–4883.

[139] Li, J., Zhang, W., Zhou, M., Kooger, R., Zhang, Y., (2013). Small molecules modulating biogenesis or processing of microRNAs with therapeutic potentials. *Curr. Med. Chem.* 20, 3604-12.

[140] Qureshi, A.T., Doyle, A., Chen, C., Coulon, D., Dasa, V., Del Piero, F., Levi, B., Monroe, W.T., Gimble, J.M., Hayes, D.J., (2015). Photoactivated miR-148b-nanoparticle conjugates improve closure of critical size mouse calvarial defects. *Acta Biomater.* 12, 166-73.

[141] Beavers, K.R., Nelson, C.E., Duvall, C.L., (2014). miRNA inhibition in tissue engineering and regenerative medicine. *Adv. Drug Deliv. Rev.* Dec 29. pii: S0169-409X(14)00311-1. doi: 10.1016/j.addr.2014.12.006. [Epub ahead of print].

[142] Dumas, J.E., Prieto, E.M., Zienkiewicz, K.J., Guda, T., Wenke, J.C., Bible, J., Holt, G.E., Guelcher, S.A., (2014). Balancing the rates of new bone formation and polymer degradation enhances healing of weight-bearing allograft/polyurethane composites in rabbit femoral defects. *Tissue Eng. Part A* 20, 115–129.

[143] Priddy, L.B., Chaudhuri, O., Stevens, H.Y., Krishnan, L., Uhrig, B.A., Willett, N.J., Guldberg, R.E., (2014). Oxidized alginate hydrogels for bone morphogenetic protein-2 delivery in long bone defects, *Acta Biomater.* 10, 4390–4399.

[144] Nguyen, M.K., Jeon, O., Krebs, M.D., Schapira, D., Alsberg, E., (2014). Sustained localized presentation of RNA interfering molecules from in situ forming hydrogels to guide 1270 stem cell osteogenic differentiation. *Biomaterials* 35, 6278–6286.

[145] Zhang, W., Wang, X., Wang, S., Zhao, J., Xu, L., Zhu, C., Zeng, D., Chen, J., Zhang, Z.B., Kaplan, D.L., (2011). The use of injectable sonication-induced silk hydrogel for VEGF165 and BMP-2 delivery for elevation of the maxillary sinus floor. *Biomaterials.* 32, 9415–9424.

[146] Xiao, W., Fu, H., Rahaman, M.N., Liu, Y., Bal, B.S., (2013). Hollow hydroxyapatite micro-spheres: a novel bioactive and osteoconductive carrier for controlled release of bone morphogenetic protein-2 in bone regeneration. *Acta Biomater.* 9, 8374–8383.

[147] Kim, M.J., Lee, B., Yang, K., Park, J., Jeon, S., Um, S.H., Kim, D.I., Im, S.G., Cho, S.W., (2013). BMP-2 peptide-functionalized nanopatterned substrates for enhanced osteogenic differentiation of human mesenchymal stem cells. *Biomaterials* 34, 1286 7236-7246.

[148] Yau, W.W., Rujitanaroj, P.O., Lam, L., Chew, S.Y., (2012). Directing stem cell fate by controlled RNA interference. *Biomaterials* 33, 2608–2628.

[149] Li, Y., Fan, L., Liu, S., Liu, W., Zhang, H., Zhou, T., Wu, D., Yang, P., Shen, L., Chen, J., (2013). The promotion of bone regeneration through positive regulation of angiogenic-osteogenic coupling using microRNA-26a. *Biomaterials* 34, 5048–5058.

[150] Murata, K., Ito, H., Yoshitomi, H., Yamamoto, K., Fukuda, A., Yoshikawa, J., Furu, M., Ishikawa, M., Shibuya, H., Matsuda, S., (2014). Inhibition of miR-92a enhances fracture healing via promoting angiogenesis in a model of stabilized fracture in young mice. *J. Bone Miner. Res.* 29, 316–326.

[151] Kosaka, N., Iguchi, H., Yoshioka, Y., Hagiwara, K., Takeshita, F., Ochiya, T., (2012). Competitive interactions of cancer cells and normal cells via secretory microRNAs. *J. Biol. Chem.* 287, 1397-1405.

[152] Suh, S., Lee, J.Y., Choi, Y.S., Chung, C.P., Park, Y.J., (2013). Peptide-mediated intracellular delivery of miRNA-29b for osteogenic stem cell differentiation. *Biomaterials* 34, 4347–4359.

[153] Deng, Y., Bi, X., Zhou, H., You, Z., Wang, Y., Gu, P., Fan, X., (2014). Repair of critical-sized bone defects with anti-miR-31-expressing bone marrow stromal stem cells and poly(glycerol sebacate) scaffolds. *Eur. Cell Mater.* 27, 13–24 (discussion 24-5).

[154] Castaño, I.M., Curtin, C.M., Shaw, G., Murphy, J.M., Duffy, G.P., O'Brien, F.J., (2014). A novel collagen-nanohydroxyapatite microRNA-activated scaffold for tissue engineering applications capable of efficient delivery of both miR-mimics and antagomiRs to human mesenchymal stem cells. *J. Control. Release* Dec 28. pii: S0168-3659(14)00831-1. doi: 10.1016/j.jconrel.2014.12.034. [Epub ahead of print].

[155] Monaghan, M., Brown, S., Schenke-Layland, K., Pandit, A., (2014). A collagen-based scaffold delivering exogenous microRNA-29B to modulate extracellular matrix remodelling. *Mol. Ther.* 22, 786–796.

[156] Mariner, P.D., Johannesen, E., Anseth, K.S., (2012). Manipulation of miRNA activity accelerates osteogenic differentiation of hMSCs in engineered 3D scaffolds. *Tissue Eng. Regen. Med.* 6, 314–324.

[157] Friedman, R.C., Farh, K.K., Burge, C.B., Bartel, D.P., (2009). Most mammalian mRNAs are conserved targets of microRNAs. *Genome Res.* 19, 92-105.

[158] Ibrahim, A.F., Weirauch, U., Thomas, M., Grunweller, A., Hartmann, R.K., Aigner, A., (2011). MicroRNA replacement therapy for miR-145 and miR-33a is efficacious in a model of colon carcinoma. *Cancer Res.*71, 5214-5224.

[159] Martelli, H., Jr., Santos, S.M., Guimarães, A.L., P‘aranaíba, L.M., Laranjeira, A.L., Coletta, R.D., Bonan, P.R., (2010). Idiopathic gingival fibromatosis: description of two cases. *Minerva Stomatol.* 59, 143–148.

[160] Damasceno, L.S., Gonçalves, Fda. S., Costa e Silva, E., Zenóbio, E.G., Souza, P.E., Horta, M.C., (2012). Stromal myofibroblasts in focal reactive overgrowths of the gingiva. *Braz. Oral Res.* 26, 373–377.

[161] Wynn, T.A., Ramalingam, T.R., (2012). Mechanisms of fibrosis: therapeutic translation for fibrotic disease. *Nat Med.* 18, 1028–1040.

[162] Guo, F., Carter, D.E., Leask, A., (2014). miR-218 regulates focal adhesion kinase-dependent TGFβ signalling in fibroblasts. *Mol. Biol. Cell.* 25(7), 1151–1158.

[163] Canady, J., Karrer, S., Fleck, M., Bosserhoff, A.K., (2013). Fibrosing connective tissue disorders of the skin: molecular similarities and distinctions. *J. Dermatol. Sci.*70, 151–158.

[164] Guo, F., Carter, D.E., Leask, A., (2011). Mechanical tension increases CCN2/CTGF expression and proliferation in gingival fibroblasts via a TGFβ-dependent mechanism. *PLoS One* 6, e19756.

[165] Mishra, R., Zhu, L., Eckert, R.L., Simonson, M.S., (2007). TGF-beta-regulated collagen type I accumulation: role of Src-based signals. *Am. J. Physiol. Cell Physiol*. 292, C1361–C1369.

[166] Guo, F., Carter, D.E., Mukhopadhyay, A., Leask, A., (2011). Gingival fibroblasts display reduced adhesion and spreading on extracellular matrix: a possible basis for scarless tissue repair. PLoS One 6, e27097.

[167] Mann, J., Mann, D.A., (2013). Epigenetic regulation of wound healing and fibrosis. *Curr. Opin. Rheumatol.* 25, 101-7.

[168] Gay, I., Cavender, A., Peto, D., Sun, Z., Speer, A., Cao, H., Amendt, B.A., (2014). Differentiation of human dental stem cells reveals a role for microRNA-218. *J. Periodontal Res.* 49, 110–120.

[169] Hidaka, H., Seki, N., Yoshino, H., Yamasaki, T., Yamada, Y., Nohata, N., Fuse, M., Nakagawa, M., Enokida, H., (2012). Tumor suppressive microRNA-1285 regulates novel molecular targets: aberrant expression and functional significance in renal cell carcinoma. *Oncotarget* 3, 44–57.

[170] Song, L., Lin, C., Gong, H., Wang, C., Liu, L., Wu, J., Tao, S., Bo Hu, B., Cheng, S-Y., Mengfeng Li, M., Jun Li, J., (2013). miR-486 sustains NF-κB activity by disrupting multiple NF-κB-negative feedback loops. *Cell Res.* 23, 274–289.

[171] Ti, D., Li, M., Fu, X., Han, W., (2014). Causes and consequences of epigenetic regulation in wound healing. *Wound Repair Regen.* 22, 305-12.

[172] Gay, I.C., Chen, S., MacDougall, M., (2007). Isolation and characterization of multipotent human periodontal ligament stem cells. *Orthod. Craniofac. Res.*10, 149–160.

[173] Huang, G.T., Gronthos, S., Shi, S., (2009). Mesenchymal stem cells derived from dental tissues vs. those from other sources: their biology and role in regenerative medicine. *J. Dent. Res.* 88, 792–806.

[174] Treves-Manusevitz, S., Hoz, L., Rachima, H., Montoya, G., Tzur, E., Vardimon, A., Sampath Narayanan, A., Amar, S., Arzate, H., Pitaru, S.,

(2013). Stem cells of the lamina propria of human oral mucosa and gingiva develop into mineralized tissues *in vivo*. *J. Clin. Periodontol.* 40, 73–81.

[175] Wang, F., Yu, M., Yan, X., Wen, Y., Zeng, Q., Yue, W., Yang, P., Pei, X., (2011). Gingiva-derived mesenchymal stem cell-mediated therapeutic approach for bone tissue regeneration. *Stem Cells Dev.* 20, 2093-102.

[176] Boiani, M., Scholer, H.R., (2005). Regulatory networks in embryo-derived pluripotent stem cells. *Nat. Rev. Mol. Cell Biol.* 6, 872–84.

[177] Lin, S.L., Kim, H., Ying, S.Y., (2008). Intron-mediated RNA interference and microRNA (miRNA). *Front. Biosci.* 13, 2216–2230.

[178] Luzi, E., Marini, F., Sala, S.C., Tognarini, I., Galli, G., Brandi, M.L., (2008). Osteogenic differentiation of human adipose tissue-derived stem cells is modulated by the miR-26a Targeting of the SMAD1transcription factor. *J. Bone Miner. Res.* 23, 287–295.

[179] Mizuno, Y., Tokuzawa, Y., Ninomiya, Y., Yagi, K., Yatsuka-Kanesaki, Y., Suda T., Fukuda, T., Katagiri, T., Kondoh, Y., Amemiya, T., Tashiro H., Okazaki Y., (2009). miR-210 promotes osteoblastic differentiation through inhibition of AcvR1b. *FEBS Lett.* 583, 2263–2268.

[180] R., Liu, W., Li, H., Yang, L., Chen, C., Xia, Z-Y, Guo L-J, Xie, H., Zhou, H-D., Wu, X-P., Luo, X-H., (2011). A Runx2/miR-3960/miR-2861 regulatory feedback loop during mouse osteoblast differentiation. *J. Biol. Chem.* 286, 12328–12339.

[181] Hassan, M.Q., Gordon, J.A.R., Beloti, M.M., Croce, C.M., van Wijnen, A.J., Stein, J.L., Stein, G.S., Lian, J.B., (2010). A network connecting Runx2, SATB2, and the miR-23a, 27a and 24-2 cluster regulates the osteoblast differentiation program. *Proc. Natl. Acad. Sci. USA*. 107, 19879-19884.

[182] Gao, J., Yang, T., Han, J., Yan, K., Qiu, X., Zhou, Y., Fan, Q., Ma, B., (2011). MicroRNA expression during osteogenic differentiation of human multipotent mesenchymal stromal cells from bone marrow. *J. Cell Biochem.* 112, 1844–1856.

[183] Zhang, Y., Xie, R.L., Croce, C.M., Stein, J.L., Lian, J.B., van Wijnen, A.J., Stein, G.S., (2011). A program of microRNAs controls osteogenic lineage progression by targeting transcription factor Runx2. *Proc. Natl. Acad. Sci. USA*. 108, 9863–9868.

[184] Lien, C.Y., Lee, O.K., Su, Y., (2007). Cbfb enhances the osteogenic differentiation of both human and mouse mesenchymal stem cells

induced by Cbfa-1 via reducing its ubiquitination-mediated degradation. *Stem Cells* 25, 1462–8.

[185] Cao, H., Wang, J., Li, X., Florez, S., Huang, Z., Venugopalan, S.R., Elangovan, S., Skobe, Z., Margolis, H.C., Martin, J.F., Amendt, B.A., (2010). MicroRNAs play a critical role in tooth development. *J. Dent. Res.* 89, 779–84.

[186] Dhanasekaran, M., Indumathi, S., Rashmi, M., Rajkumar, J.S., Sudarsanam, D., (2012). Unravelling the retention of proliferation and differentiation potency in extensive culture of human subcutaneous fat-derived mesenchymal stem cells in different media. *Cell Prolif.* 45, 516–26.

[187] Kawanabe, N., Murata, S., Fukushima, H., Ishihara, Y., Yanagita, T., Yanagita, E., Ono, M., Kurosaka, H., Kamioka, H., Itoh, T., Kuboki, T., Yamashiro, T., (2012). Stage-specific embryonic antigen-4 identifies human dental pulp stem cells. *Exp. Cell Res.* 318, 453–63.

[188] Atari, M., Barajas, M., Hernandez-Alfaro, F., Gil, C., Fabregat, M., Ferres Padro, E., Giner, L., Casals, N., (2011). Isolation of pluripotent stem cells from human third molar dental pulp. *Histol. Histopathol.* 26, 1057–70.

[189] Seo, B.M., Miura, M., Gronthos, S., Bartold, P.M., Batouli, S., Brahim, J., Young, M., Robey, P.G., Wang, C.Y., Shi, S., (2004). Investigation of multipotent postnatal stem cells from human periodontal ligament. *Lancet* 364, 149–55.

[190] Nagatomo, K., Komaki, M., Sekiya, I., Sakaguchi, Y., Noguchi, K., Oda, S., Muneta, T., Ishikawa, I., (2006). Stem cell properties of human periodontal ligament cells. *J. Periodontal Res.* 41, 303–310.

[191] Lian, J.B., Javed, A., Zaidi, S.K., Lengner, C., Montecino, M., van Wijnen, A.J., Stein, J.L., Stein, G.S., (2004). Regulatory controls for osteoblast growth and differentiation: role of Runx/Cbfa/AML factors. *Crit. Rev. Eukaryot. Gene Expr.* 14, 1–41.

[192] Lee, M.K., DeConde, A.S., Lee, M., Walthers, C.M., Sepahdari, A.R., Elashoff, D., Grogan, T., Bezouglaia, O., Tetradis, S., St. John, M., Aghaloo, T., (2015). Biomimetic scaffolds facilitate healing of critical-sized segmental mandibular defects. *Am. J. Otolaryngol.* 36, 1-6.

[193] Zhao, S., Zhang, J., Zhu, M., Zhang, Y., Liu, Z., Tao, C., Zhu, Y., Zhang, C., (2015). Three-dimensional printed strontium-containing mesoporous bioactive glass scaffolds for repairing rat critical-sized calvarial defects. *Acta Biomater.* 12, 270-80.

[194] Shim, J.H., Yoon, M.C., Jeong, C.M., Jang, J., Jeong, S.I., Cho, D.W., Huh, J.B., (2014). Efficacy of rhBMP-2 loaded PCL/PLGA/β-TCP guided bone regeneration membrane fabricated by 3D printing technology for reconstruction of calvaria defects in rabbit. *Biomed Mater.* 9, 065006. doi: 10.1088/1748-6041/9/6/065006.
[195] Shim, J.H., Kim, S.E., Park, J.Y., Kundu, J., Kim, S.W., Kang, S.S., Cho, D.W., (2014). Three-dimensional printing of rhBMP-2-loaded scaffolds with long-term delivery for enhanced bone regeneration in a rabbit diaphyseal defect. *Tissue Eng Part A*. 20, 1980-92.
[196] Inzana, J.A., Olvera, D., Fuller, S.M., Kelly, J.P., Graeve, O.A., Schwarz, E.M., Kates, S.L., Awad, H.A., (2014). 3D printing of composite calcium phosphate and collagen scaffolds for bone regeneration. *Biomaterials* 35, 4026-34.
[197] Oryan, A., Alidadi, S., Moshiri, A., Maffulli, N., (2014). Bone regenerative medicine: classic options, novel strategies, and future directions. *J. Orthop. Surg. Res.* 9, 18. doi: 10.1186/1749-799X-9-18.
[198] O'Brien, C.M., Holmes, B., Faucett, S., Zhang, L.G., (2014). Three-Dimensional Printing of nanomaterial scaffolds for complex tissue regeneration. *Tissue Eng Part B Rev.* Sep 16. [Epub ahead of print].
[199] Wu, C., Luo, Y., Cuniberti, G., Xiao, Y., Gelinsky, M., (2011). Three-dimensional printing of hierarchical and tough mesoporous bioactive glass scaffolds with a controllable pore architecture, excellent mechanical strength and mineralization ability. *Acta Biomater.* 7, 2644-2650.

Index

#

3D apatite scaffolds, 40
3D material constructs, 36
3D printing, x, 8, 61, 62, 63, 64, 65, 88
3D-printed biomimetic scaffolds, 61

A

access, 14
acid, 3, 6, 26, 43, 62, 63, 70
adhesion, 3, 23, 28, 39, 54, 55, 75, 85
adipose, 27, 37, 38, 40, 51, 61, 86
adipose tissue, 27, 38, 86
adult stem cells, 1, 38
adults, 54
advancement, 64
adverse effects, 12
age, 33, 57, 58, 59
aggregation, 9
aluminium, 11
alveolar bone, 6, 12
ameloblastin, 9
amelogenin, 9
amino, 39, 77
amino acid(s), 39, 77
androgen, 10
angiogenesis, 2, 9, 49, 50, 52, 79, 80, 81, 83
anisotropy, 36
antagomiRNAs, 53, 54
antibody, 18, 34, 58
antigen, 12, 87
antioxidant, 23
apoptosis, 53, 56
assessment, 77
attachment, 9, 15, 34, 44, 75
Autografts, 2, 11, 64

B

bacterial infection, 50
banking, 24
barrier membranes, ix, 6, 15
barriers, 8
beneficial effect, 20, 53
Bible, 83
bilayered scaffold, 39
binder solution, 63
bioactive agents, 36
Bioactivity, 64
bioceramics, 46
biocompatibility, 3, 11, 44, 45, 46, 63
biodegradability, 64
biodegradable, 2, 12, 25, 44, 45, 65
biodiversity, 44
biological activity, 52
biological processes, 56
biological systems, 44
biomarkers, v, 17, 20, 34, 49, 74

biomaterials, vii, 1, 3, 10, 15, 25, 27, 28, 29, 30, 31, 38, 39, 40, 43, 44, 45, 62, 64, 67, 70, 71, 74, 75, 77, 80
biomedical applications, ix, 1, 2, 45
biomimetic, x, 2, 8, 21, 29, 44, 61
biomimetic scaffolds, 2, 29, 44
biomolecules, 34
biopolymers, 45
biopsy, 74
bioreactors, 28
bioresorbable, 44
bonding, 47
bone, vii, ix, x, 2, 3, 5, 6, 7, 8, 9, 10, 11, 12, 13, 14, 15, 18, 19, 21, 22, 23, 24, 27, 30, 34, 35, 37, 39, 40, 41, 43, 44, 46, 47, 51, 52, 54, 57, 58, 61, 62, 63, 64, 69, 70, 71, 72, 73, 74, 77, 78, 79, 80, 83, 84, 86, 88
bone form, x, 3, 14, 19, 22, 24, 40, 44, 52, 61, 62, 83
bone growth, 22, 36
bone marrow, 14, 18, 22, 24, 27, 37, 39, 52, 57, 58, 74, 84, 86
bone mass, 18
bone mineral, 10, 18, 71
bone regeneration, 10, 15, 22, 23, 24, 35, 36, 40, 44, 47, 52, 54, 61, 62, 63, 64, 70, 71, 74, 78, 80, 83, 88
bone resorption, 19, 73
bones, 63
branching, 79
breakdown, 23
brittleness, 65
building blocks, 39, 44

C

Ca^{2+}, 29
calcium, 22, 23, 39, 43, 46, 58, 63, 78, 79, 88
calcium phosphate, 22, 23, 39, 43, 46, 63, 78, 79, 88
calvaria, 88
calvarium, 51
cancer, 55, 81, 84
cancer cells, 55, 84
candidates, 24
CaP, 46
carcinoma, 84
cartilage, 17, 19, 30, 38, 39, 73
cascades, 28, 59
casting, 47, 79
CCN2/CTGF, 73, 85
cell based therapy, 14
cell biology, 1, 43
cell culture, ix, 1, 18, 22, 26, 40, 44, 74
cell differentiation, 1, 2, 3, 6, 28, 29, 43, 54, 58, 59, 84
cell fate, 25, 83
cell invasion, 44
cell line, 14, 21, 28, 57, 59
cell movement, 26
cell phenotype, ix, 2, 56, 57
Cell therapy, 31
cell/gene therapy, 7
cell-signalling, 2, 56
Cementoblast differentiation, 7
ceramic, 46, 79
challenges, 27, 46, 47, 64
chemical(s), 7, 24, 27, 28, 40, 47
chemokines, 56
chitosan, 11, 12, 40, 43, 72, 78
chitosan-based hydrogels, 12
chondrocyte, 17, 20
circulation, 18, 46
classes, 44
clinical application, vii, ix, x, 3, 6, 22, 24, 25, 30, 33, 38, 45, 67, 69, 76
clinical attachment, 9
clinical trials, 9, 11, 14, 18, 30, 44
closure, 50, 51, 82
coatings, x, 2, 40
coding, x, 49, 51, 55
collagen, 3, 13, 18, 22, 27, 29, 35, 36, 39, 40, 43, 44, 45, 47, 53, 55, 62, 63, 72, 77, 79, 84, 85, 88
colon, 84
combined effect, 29, 30
communication, 7, 18, 70
complex interactions, 64
complexity, 29

complications, 14, 49, 50, 80
composites, 40, 43, 63, 83
composition, 2, 7, 9, 28, 29, 54
computer, 2
Concise, 74
connective tissue, 8, 13, 19, 36, 54, 72, 85
consensus, 6, 13, 70, 71, 72
construction, 38, 39, 43, 64
control group, 34
controlled studies, 37
convergence, 43
coordination, vii, 54, 59
correlation, 58
cost, 6, 30
covering, 11, 14
CSD, 52
CT, 35
cues, 3, 7, 28, 30, 49, 76
culture, 7, 8, 10, 18, 26, 29, 30, 38, 59, 74, 75, 87
culture conditions, 38
current limit, 1
cycles, 29, 73
cytocompatibility, 63
cytokines, 41, 49, 50, 56
cytoskeleton, 28, 29
cytotoxicity, 53

D

debridement, 10, 11, 15
decision-making process, 51
defect site, 11
defects, vii, 7, 8, 10, 11, 13, 15, 22, 35, 39, 40, 44, 45, 46, 47, 52, 61, 62, 63, 64, 71, 72, 79, 82, 83, 84, 87, 88
deficiencies, 13
deficit, 2
deformation, 44
degradation, 2, 12, 26, 34, 35, 40, 45, 49, 83, 87
degradation mechanism, 26
degradation rate, 12
delivery platforms, 7
demineralised bone matrix, 15
dental apical papilla, 7, 70
dental caries, 8
dental stem cells, 55, 57, 85
deposition, 29, 34
deposits, 58, 59
depth, 15
desorption, 80
detachment, 45, 47
diabetes, 38, 81
diabetic retinopathy, 82
diagnostic markers, 50
direct action, 10
diseases, 2, 8, 18, 28, 30, 37, 45, 50, 51, 54, 56
distribution, 27, 39
divergence, 36
diversity, 24, 26, 39, 51, 55
DNA, 12, 20, 56
dogs, 37
down-regulation, 20, 40, 52, 59
drug delivery, 3, 7, 27, 64
drug release, 3
drugs, 36, 56, 81
DSC, 57

E

E-cadherin, 41
ECM, ix, 1, 2, 21, 26, 29, 40, 44, 54, 59, 67
electrospinning, 44
electrospun matrices, 26, 44
ELISA, 35
elucidation, 24, 64
embryonic stem cells, 30, 38, 41, 57, 58
enamel, 7, 9, 11, 13, 71
encapsulation, 27
endoderm, 58
endothelial cells, 17, 46, 47
endothelium, 45, 46, 47
engineering, viii, 2, 3, 7, 8, 10, 14, 15, 22, 23, 24, 25, 26, 28, 29, 30, 35, 36, 40, 43, 44, 45, 47, 53, 54, 64, 70, 74, 77, 79, 80
environment, ix, 7, 23, 25, 26, 28, 29, 30, 44, 51, 71
environmental conditions, 30

environmental cues, 30
Epigenetic mechanisms, 56
epigenetics, 56
epithelial cells, 9
epithelium, 6
epitopes, 33
ethical issues, 18
ethylene, 26, 27
ethylene glycol, 26, 27
evidence, 9, 13, 38, 46, 71
evolution, 28, 44, 55, 56
ex vivo culture, 30
excitability, 82
expertise, 3
exposure, 12, 51
extracellular matrices, ix, 1, 75
extracellular matrix, 3, 5, 23, 25, 36, 74, 76, 84, 85
Extracellular vesicles, 1, 69
extrusion, 36, 77

F

fabrication, 2, 34, 40, 43, 61, 63, 73, 78
fat, 61, 81, 87
FDA, 44
FDI, 45
fibers, 77
fibrin, x, 2, 11, 43
fibroblast(s), 10, 21, 23, 30, 35, 38, 39, 49, 50, 54, 55, 56, 71, 74, 80, 81, 85
fibroblast growth factor, 35
fibrosis, 20, 49, 55, 84, 85
fillers, 8
films, 40
flap surgery, 11, 15
flexibility, 26, 35
fluid, 76
follicle, 7
force, 28
formation, 5, 6, 9, 12, 19, 22, 23, 25, 26, 29, 34, 39, 40, 46, 47, 56, 59, 62, 63, 64
fractures, 18, 52, 64
fusion, 1, 44, 78

G

gallium, 11
gel, 12, 22
gelation, 12, 26, 72
gene delivery, 8, 31, 33
gene expression, x, 9, 21, 28, 35, 37, 49, 50, 51, 56, 62, 63
gene pool, 43
gene regulation, 54
gene therapy, 7, 8, 15, 30, 38, 53, 64
genes, 29, 43, 51, 53, 55, 56, 58, 69
genome, 19
geometry, 75
germ line, 33
gingivae, 14, 54, 55, 57
gingival, 5, 13, 30, 54, 55, 56, 58, 72, 84, 85
glasses, 43
glucose, 20, 73
glutathione, 10, 71
glycerol, 84
grading, 71
grafting materials, ix, 6, 10, 11, 64
growth, vii, ix, 1, 2, 6, 7, 8, 9, 10, 15, 19, 20, 24, 26, 28, 29, 34, 35, 36, 41, 44, 46, 49, 52, 55, 56, 64, 67, 70, 75, 76, 80, 87
growth factor(s), vii, ix, 1, 2, 6, 7, 8, 9, 10, 15, 19, 29, 34, 35, 36, 41, 44, 46, 49, 52, 55, 56, 64, 67, 76, 80
guidance, 2

H

HAP, 39, 40
hard tissues, 43
harvesting, 14, 17
HE, 6
healing, vii, 10, 14, 15, 22, 23, 49, 50, 51, 52, 56, 61, 62, 63, 64, 71, 74, 81, 82, 83, 87
health, 8, 9
heterogeneity, 13, 38
histamine, 23, 74
histology, 40

histone, 56
homeostasis, 33
hormone(s), 18, 41
horses, 37
host, 6, 9, 39, 44, 45, 46, 62
hub, 19
human, 8, 9, 10, 11, 15, 17, 23, 30, 34, 35, 44, 50, 51, 53, 57, 58, 59, 60, 62, 69, 70, 71, 73, 74, 76, 79, 83, 84, 85, 86, 87
human subjects, 8
hybrid, 39
hydrogels, v, ix, 2, 3, 11, 12, 25, 26, 27, 34, 72, 74, 75, 79, 80, 83
hydroxyapatite, 39, 43, 70, 77, 83
hypothesis, 22, 27, 55

I

ideal, 24, 65
identity, 18
immune response, 38
immunogenicity, 17, 18
immunomodulatory, 38
implants, 7, 13, 18, 44, 63
in vitro, 2, 9, 10, 22, 23, 27, 28, 30, 34, 35, 36, 43, 47, 51, 52, 63, 71, 75, 77
in vitro environment, 28
in vivo, 2, 10, 11, 22, 28, 30, 33, 34, 35, 36, 38, 40, 43, 44, 45, 46, 47, 50, 51, 52, 62, 67, 74, 77, 86
individuals, 2
inducer, 44
induction, 5, 17, 23, 35, 40, 43, 44, 52, 54, 55, 56, 57, 62
infection, 52, 64
inflammation, ix, 6, 24, 25, 50, 82
inflammatory disease, 31
inguinal, 61
inhibition, 26, 29, 41, 52, 53, 56, 59, 82, 86
inhibitor, 41, 52
injury, 17, 54, 56
insertion, 46
insulin, 82
insulin resistance, 82
integration, 6, 26, 39, 45, 46, 47, 53
integrin, 75
interface, 36
interference, 44, 53, 83, 86
interferons, 41
interphase, 18
intrabony defect fill, 9
investment, 67
issues, 38

K

keratinocyte, 50, 80
keratinocytes, 50
kidney, 82
kinetics, 7, 35, 45

L

lactic acid, 43
lasers, ix, 6
lead, 36, 37, 40, 64
legal issues, 38
leptin, 41
lesions, 37
leucine, 9
lifetime, 52
ligament, 5, 6, 7, 9, 10, 11, 12, 21, 34, 57, 58, 72, 85, 87
ligand, 33
light, 26
lithium, 34
loaded scaffolds, 8, 15, 88
localization, 26, 41, 78
low risk, 5
Luo, 86, 88

M

macromolecules, ix, 1
macrophages, 63
macropores, 62
magnitude, 34
majority, 43
management, 10, 11, 13, 18, 28, 31

mandible, 35, 47
manipulation, ix, 1, 19, 50, 53
manufacturing, 2
marrow, 5, 22, 24, 27, 38, 39, 57, 58, 59, 81
Marx, 77
mass, 18, 35
mass spectrometry, 35
materials, vii, ix, 6, 9, 10, 11, 22, 26, 29, 43, 44, 64, 65, 67, 70, 72, 78
matrix, vii, ix, 1, 2, 5, 7, 9, 10, 11, 13, 15, 18, 22, 23, 26, 29, 30, 44, 71, 72
maxillary sinus, 83
mechanical cue, 27
mechanical properties, 30, 63
mechanical stress, 7, 18, 55
mechanical stretching, 29, 76
mechano-transduction, 18
media, 17, 22, 87
medical, viii, 3, 71
medicine, ix, 1, 2, 33, 37, 38, 44, 77, 78
membranes, ix, 6, 10, 15, 62
memory, 75
mesenchymal stem cells, 1, 5, 14, 17, 18, 30, 50, 52, 53, 59, 69, 70, 73, 75, 76, 78, 79, 83, 84, 86, 87
mesenchyme, 14
mesoderm, 58
mesoporous bioactive glass scaffolds, 62, 87, 88
meta-analysis, 11, 72
metabolic responses, 23
metabolism, 18, 19
meth, 34
methylation, 56
mice, 22, 24, 41, 49, 50, 51, 81, 82, 83
microenvironments, 75
microfabrication, 8
microgels, 27
microparticles, 3, 34
microRNA(s), 21, 24, 49, 57, 80, 81, 82, 83, 84, 85, 86
microspheres, 35, 76
microvascular networks, 46, 79
migration, 26, 49, 50, 56, 81
mimicry, 21, 50
mineralization, 3, 19, 27, 34, 35, 39, 40, 59, 65, 88
miRNA mimics, 53
MiRNA profiles, 59
miRNA therapeutics, 53
models, 36, 39, 50, 55
modifications, 56
molecular biology, vii, ix, 1, 67
Molecular redundancy, 8
molecules, x, 2, 5, 6, 14, 19, 24, 36, 37, 40, 49, 50, 51, 53, 82, 83
monolayer, 7, 53, 75
monomers, 36
morbidity, 1, 2, 5, 9, 13, 14, 17, 52, 64
morphogenesis, 25, 43, 58, 80
morphology, 10, 15, 18, 22, 23, 36
mortality, 9, 54
moulding, 46
mRNA(s), x, 20, 49, 51, 52, 55, 58, 84
mucosa, 86
multiple isoforms, 8, 14
Multiple recession defects, 13
multipotent, 24, 28, 30, 33, 38, 85, 86, 87
musculoskeletal, 30, 33, 76
musculoskeletal system, 30
mutation, 33
myofibroblasts, 54, 55, 56, 84

N

nanoagents, 64
nanoclay, 39, 77
nanoformulated miRNA, 51
nanohydroxyapatite, 6, 53, 70, 84
nanomaterials, 64
nanoparticles, 51, 81
nanotechnology, vii, 1, 50, 67
natural polymers, 43
neovascularization, 17
neurons, 81
neuropathic pain, 82
nicotine, 10, 71
nitric oxide, 17
norbornene, 26, 74
normal development, 25

nucleic acid, 36
nucleus, 41
nutrients, 45
nutrition, 45, 46

O

opportunities, 5, 18, 35
optimization, 40
oral cavity, 1, 5, 14, 21, 54, 67, 70
oral diseases, 39
orchestration, 43
organ(s), 1, 14, 20, 23, 26, 27, 36, 38, 54, 56, 80
osteoarthritis, 30
osteoblast differentiation, 58, 59, 60, 86
osteocalcin, 29, 34, 35, 63
osteocyte, 18, 19, 73
Osteogenesis, 79
osteogenic cells, 64
osteoinductive/osteoconductive, 52
osteopontin, 29, 34
osteoporosis, 18
overlap, 51, 59
oxidative stress, 10, 25
oxygen, 26, 45, 46

P

pain, 23
parallel, 57
patents, 8
pathogenesis, 82
pathology, 2
pathophysiological, 50, 51
pathways, 5, 19, 24, 29, 41, 44, 50, 51, 56, 58
PDGFR, 41
PDL, 58
peptide(s), ix, 6, 8, 9, 10, 26, 75, 83
perfusion, 46, 47, 80
perinatal, 24
periodontal, vii, ix, 5, 6, 7, 8, 9, 10, 11, 12, 13, 14, 15, 20, 21, 22, 34, 57, 58, 67, 70, 71, 72, 85, 87
periodontal disease, 5, 8, 34
periodontal regeneration, vii, ix, 5, 6, 8, 9, 10, 11, 13, 20, 22, 67, 70, 71
periodontitis, 6, 7, 8
periosteal cell sheets, 21, 22
periosteum, 21, 22, 23, 24, 73, 74
Periostin, 23
peripheral blood, 81
peripheral blood mononuclear cell, 81
permit, 75
pH, 28
phenotype(s), ix, 2, 29, 30, 38, 39, 56, 57, 58
phenytoin, 23, 74
phosphate, 9, 22, 23, 39, 43, 45, 46, 47, 63, 78, 79, 88
phosphorylation, 20, 29, 41
photoclick hydrogels, 26
photolithography, 2, 46
physical characteristics, 62
physical environment, 27
physical properties, 34
Physiological, 43
PI3K, 41
plaque, 5
plasticity, 57, 58
platform, 35, 39, 45, 51, 53
pluripotency, 3, 41, 58
polyesters, 43
polymer(s), 23, 25, 28, 35, 43, 44, 83
polymer systems, 25
polymerization, 69
polysaccharides, 40
polyurethane, 44, 65, 78, 83
polyurethane foam, 65
polyvinyl alcohol, 65
population, 24, 27, 58
pore architecture, 65, 88
porosity, 39, 62
predictability, vii, 15
premolars, 13
preparation, 14, 64, 78

prevention, 49
principles, vii, ix, 1, 6, 10, 44, 56
prior knowledge, 21
progenitor cells, 2, 5, 20, 21, 22, 24, 25, 30, 38, 46, 49, 70, 72, 74, 81
prognosis, 10
programming, 41
pro-inflammatory, 82
proliferation, ix, 1, 2, 9, 12, 27, 30, 33, 37, 39, 41, 43, 50, 53, 55, 56, 62, 78, 85, 87
protein family, 41
proteins, ix, 1, 8, 9, 10, 15, 19, 29, 52, 53, 76
prototype, 33
pulp, 7, 57, 58, 87
purity, 18
PVA, 65

Q

quality of life, 2

R

reactions, 26
reagents, 40
recession, 13
reconstruction, 6, 7, 47, 49, 70, 88
redundancy, 8, 50
regenerate, ix, 1, 7, 22, 70
regeneration, vii, viii, ix, 1, 2, 5, 6, 7, 8, 9, 10, 11, 13, 14, 15, 20, 21, 22, 23, 24, 25, 27, 29, 30, 34, 35, 36, 38, 39, 40, 44, 46, 47, 51, 52, 54, 57, 61, 62, 63, 64, 67, 70, 71, 72, 73, 74, 76, 78, 80, 83, 86, 88
regenerative biology, 10, 28
regenerative capacity, 12, 24, 73
regenerative medicine, vii, ix, 1, 2, 3, 5, 14, 25, 26, 27, 28, 33, 34, 36, 38, 39, 43, 44, 45, 46, 51, 67, 69, 73, 74, 76, 78, 82, 85, 88
regenerative Medicine/Dentistry., viii, 3, 24
regenerative surgical procedures, vii, 15
regulatory bodies, 37
rejection, 5, 64
Release kinetics, 35
relevance, 14, 38, 74
remodelling, 3, 18, 19, 24, 54, 73, 84
renal cell carcinoma, 85
repair, vii, ix, 1, 2, 7, 10, 17, 20, 21, 23, 26, 30, 34, 38, 40, 46, 50, 52, 54, 55, 56, 61, 62, 64, 74, 77, 79, 82, 85
replication, 12, 28
repression, 60
reproduction, 38
requirements, 6, 14, 67
researchers, 67
resolution, ix, 6, 36
response, 8, 10, 11, 12, 18, 21, 23, 29, 34, 35, 40, 41, 43, 50, 52, 54, 55, 56, 62, 63, 76, 81
restoration, 6, 21, 33
restrictions, 25
rheumatoid arthritis, 30
risk, 50, 64
RNA(s), x, 40, 49, 50, 53, 56, 57, 81, 83, 86
root, 6, 9, 10, 13, 14, 15, 72

S

safety, 6, 30, 39, 45
scaffold coatings, x, 2
scaffolds, ix, x, 1, 2, 3, 5, 6, 7, 8, 22, 23, 26, 27, 29, 30, 35, 39, 40, 43, 44, 45, 46, 47, 51, 52, 53, 61, 62, 63, 64, 69, 70, 77, 78, 79, 80, 84, 87, 88
science, vii, ix, 1, 8, 43, 67
scientific knowledge, 38
sclerostin, 18, 19, 34, 73
scope, 7, 10, 21, 24, 30, 52, 56
secrete, 37
secretion, 7, 18, 70
seeding, 26, 40
self-repair, 2
senescence, 20, 56, 73
sensitivity, 2, 15, 47
sequencing, 5
shear, 29, 76
sheep, 79

showing, 9, 40, 49
side effects, 35, 50
signal transduction, 44, 56
signalling, ix, 1, 2, 5, 7, 19, 24, 28, 29, 34, 41, 50, 55, 56, 57, 59, 76, 85
signals, 5, 8, 12, 14, 18, 19, 36, 38, 41, 85
silk, 39, 45, 77, 79, 83
silver, 51
simulation, 46
sintering, 65
skin, 17, 36, 49, 54, 85
slow delivery system, 62
smart biomaterial, 21, 25, 67
smoking, 10
smooth muscle, 54
solution, 62, 63
somatic cell, 38
spatiotemporal release kinetics, 7
species, 37
spliced membrane, 15
stability, 15, 38
state(s), 33, 59
stem cell differentiation, 29, 59, 84
stem cells, ix, 1, 5, 8, 14, 17, 18, 20, 26, 27, 28, 30, 33, 37, 38, 40, 41, 49, 50, 51, 52, 53, 55, 57, 58, 59, 60, 61, 67, 69, 70, 73, 75, 76, 77, 78, 79, 83, 84, 85, 86, 87
stimulation, 44, 57, 59, 69, 78
stress, 10, 29, 76
stretching, 29, 76
stroke, 38
stroma, 22
stromal cells, 22, 24, 39, 58, 63, 86
strontium, 62, 87
structure, 2, 9, 26, 36, 44, 45, 62
substitutes, 6, 11, 27, 63, 64
substrate(s), ix, 1, 3, 23, 26, 28, 29, 75, 83
Sun, 70, 77, 85
suppression, 19
surface chemistry, 28
surface tension, 63
survival, 46
susceptibility, 8, 53, 67
syndrome, 50, 82
synthesis, x, 7, 10, 23, 36, 44, 45
Synthetic ECMs, 26

T

target, x, 6, 49, 50, 51, 54, 58, 80, 81
techniques, 8, 15, 28, 36, 43, 46, 64, 77
technologies, ix, 5, 7, 44, 64
technology, vii, ix, 1, 2, 8, 15, 23, 28, 29, 36, 51, 64, 67, 88
teeth, 5, 6, 7, 8, 10, 13
temperature, 63, 65
tension, 85
testosterone, 23
TGF, 7, 18, 19, 22, 33, 54, 55, 56, 74, 76, 85
therapeutic agents, 51, 52, 53
therapeutic approaches, 47
therapeutic goal, 8
therapeutic interventions, ix, 1
therapeutic targets, 50, 51
therapeutics, 2, 6, 30, 53, 56, 67, 70, 76
therapy, ix, 2, 5, 6, 7, 8, 10, 11, 14, 15, 22, 24, 25, 27, 28, 30, 31, 37, 38, 53, 57, 67, 81, 84
thermal inkjet printing, 63
thermal treatment, 63
third molar(s), 57, 87
thrombosis, 80
tissue engineering, vii, viii, x, 1, 2, 3, 7, 8, 10, 14, 15, 21, 24, 25, 26, 28, 30, 33, 34, 36, 37, 38, 39, 40, 43, 44, 45, 46, 47, 52, 53, 57, 64, 65, 67, 69, 70, 74, 76, 77, 78, 79, 82, 84
tissue homeostasis, 27
TNF, 50
tooth, 5, 6, 8, 10, 34, 87
transcription, 29, 41, 57, 58, 59, 86
transcription factors, 57, 59
transcriptional regulation, 43
transducer, 41
transduction, 18
transfection, 49, 53
transforming growth factor, 7
translation, 25, 52, 67, 84
translocation, 41

transmission, 2, 53, 64
transplantation, 8, 12
transport, 26
transportation, 14, 38
trauma, 2, 46
treatment, 2, 5, 8, 10, 11, 13, 14, 15, 20, 30, 35, 50, 53, 67, 71, 72, 81, 82
treatment methods, 5
trial, 47, 72
triggers, 18
turnover, 21
type 2 diabetes, 81, 82
tyrosine, 41

U

umbilical cord, 18, 38, 73
uniform, 62
unique features, 24
untranslated regions, 51
urea, 12
USA, 76, 79, 80, 86
UV, 26
UV light, 26

V

validation, 51
variables, 8, 67
vascular bundle, 46
vascularization, 45, 46, 79, 80
vasculature, 5, 44, 45, 46, 62
vehicles, 14
vehicular microcapsules, 8, 15
vein, 47
versatility, 39, 45, 47
vessels, 46
viscosity, 63
volumetric collagen, 63

W

water, 25, 45
Wnt signalling, 29, 34, 76
workers, viii
wound healing, 8, 10, 11, 12, 15, 17, 23, 49, 50, 51, 56, 80, 81, 85

X

xenografts, 2, 64

Y

yield, 38, 43